THE **COMPLETE IDIOT'S GUIDE®** TO

Losing 20 Pounds in 2 Months

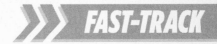
FAST-TRACK

by Wendy Watkins

ALPHA
A member of Penguin Group (USA) Inc.

ALPHA BOOKS

Published by Penguin Group (USA) Inc.

Penguin Group (USA) Inc., 375 Hudson Street, New York, New York 10014, USA • Penguin Group (Canada), 90 Eglinton Avenue East, Suite 700, Toronto, Ontario M4P 2Y3, Canada (a division of Pearson Penguin Canada Inc.) • Penguin Books Ltd., 80 Strand, London WC2R 0RL, England • Penguin Ireland, 25 St. Stephen's Green, Dublin 2, Ireland (a division of Penguin Books Ltd.) • Penguin Group (Australia), 250 Camberwell Road, Camberwell, Victoria 3124, Australia (a division of Pearson Australia Group Pty. Ltd.) • Penguin Books India Pvt. Ltd., 11 Community Centre, Panchsheel Park, New Delhi—110 017, India • Penguin Group (NZ), 67 Apollo Drive, Rosedale, North Shore, Auckland 1311, New Zealand (a division of Pearson New Zealand Ltd.) • Penguin Books (South Africa) (Pty.) Ltd., 24 Sturdee Avenue, Rosebank, Johannesburg 2196, South Africa • Penguin Books Ltd., Registered Offices: 80 Strand, London WC2R 0RL, England

Copyright © 2013 by Penguin Group (USA) Inc.

International Standard Book Number: 978-1-61564-249-6
Library of Congress Catalog Card Number: 2012947184

15 14 13   8 7 6 5 4 3 2 1

Interpretation of the printing code: The rightmost number of the first series of numbers is the year of the book's printing; the rightmost number of the second series of numbers is the number of the book's printing. For example, a printing code of 13-1 shows that the first printing occurred in 2013.

Printed in the United States of America

Note: This publication contains the opinions and ideas of its author. It is intended to provide helpful and informative material on the subject matter covered. It is sold with the understanding that the author and publisher are not engaged in rendering professional services in the book. If the reader requires personal assistance or advice, a competent professional should be consulted.

The author and publisher specifically disclaim any responsibility for any liability, loss, or risk, personal or otherwise, which is incurred as a consequence, directly or indirectly, of the use and application of any of the contents of this book.

Most Alpha books are available at special quantity discounts for bulk purchases for sales promotions, premiums, fund-raising, or educational use. Special books, or book excerpts, can also be created to fit specific needs. For details, write: Special Markets, Alpha Books, 375 Hudson Street, New York, NY 10014.

Publisher: *Mike Sanders*
Executive Managing Editor: *Billy Fields*
Senior Acquisitions Editor: *Tom Stevens*
Senior Development Editor: *Christy Wagner*
Senior Production Editor: *Kayla Dugger*

Cover Designer: *William Thomas*
Book Designers: *William Thomas and Rebecca Batchelor*
Indexer: *Heather McNeill*
Layout: *Ayanna Lacey*
Proofreader: *Cate Schwenk*

Contents

Introduction

"How did *that* happen?"

Have you ever stepped on the scale and been surprised at the number glaring back at you? Or attempted to zip up a favorite pair of jeans and found they didn't fit the way they used to? You're not alone.

If you need to lose a few pounds quickly, you've come to the right place. The weight-loss program I share in this book helps you melt off extra pounds in 2 months so you can get back in those jeans. Whether you're losing weight for a special event or just because you want a leaner version of you, this plan helps get the scale moving in the right direction. And then, when you reach your weight-loss goal, it helps you keep off those pounds—for life.

Using the diet I share in this book, you can design a meal plan filled with foods you enjoy in the proper amounts. Then, you can use the plan to ramp up your weight loss by burning more calories not only through exercise but also during your regular everyday activities. Along the way, you learn to tweak the plan to make it fit your life and your unique needs.

You *can* lose 20 pounds in 2 months. In this book, I show you how.

How This Book Is Organized

I've set up this book to make it as easy as possible for you to use.

In **Chapters 1 and 2,** I help you get organized to start your diet, including getting your kitchen outfitted with the right tools and your mind outfitted with the right mind-set.

In **Chapter 3,** I show you how to outline your specific plan, based on your current weight and activity level. Then you create a balanced meal plan from a variety of different foods that will keep you feeling satisfied as the weight comes off.

In **Chapter 4,** you put your plan in action, with emphasis on preparing your meals in advance so you don't end up making an emergency trip to the fast-food drive-thru. You also explore strategies to stay on your diet when temptations pop up.

In **Chapter 5,** I discuss the importance of NEAT (nonexercise activity thermogenesis) calories—the number of calories you burn not through exercise, but as you go about your daily life—when it comes to weight loss and share strategies to boost your NEAT quotient.

Chapters 6 and 7 include specially designed workouts to help rev up your metabolism so you burn even more calories. I also show you how to use a combination of resistance training and cardio workouts to build your body's fat-burning furnace to become leaner and stronger.

Chapters 8 and 9 help you deal with the inevitable challenges that arise when you're dieting, whether you're battling cravings and emotional eating or socializing with co-workers, family, or friends who aren't watching their weight.

In case you're dieting for a special event, **Chapter 10** offers some last-minute tips to rev up your fat loss, and **Chapter 11** helps you come up with a strategy for keeping the weight off.

At the back of the book, I've included a glossary of terms and further resources so you can make your diet and workout plan more your own.

Extras

Throughout the book, I've included brief bright ideas that point out shortcuts and cautions along the way. Here's what to look for:

 DANGER ZONE

These sidebars offer warnings about pitfalls that can occur, potentially delaying your progress.

DEFINITION

These sidebars explain diet-related terms you might not be familiar with.

TRY THIS!

These sidebars provide quick tips to make your diet plan even more effective.

Acknowledgments

Thanks to my business partner, Sean Soucy, who helped keep my in-person clients in shape when I was busy writing this book, and also thanks to agent Marilyn Allen, for making it possible for me present this plan to clients far beyond the walls of my gym. Registered dietitian (and client!) Rosemary Delano-Merritt, MEd, RD, LD, also contributed her much-appreciated expertise in double-checking the diet program.

And a huge thank you goes to my personal training clients, who inspire me every day with their positive attitudes and devotion to fitness.

Special Thanks to the Technical Reviewer

The Complete Idiot's Guide to Losing 20 Pounds in 2 Months Fast-Track was reviewed by an expert who double-checked the accuracy of what you'll learn here, to help us ensure that this book gives you everything you need to know to lose weight quickly and safely—and keep it off. Special thanks are extended to Rosemary Delano-Merritt, MEd, RD, LD.

Rosemary is owner of RDMaine, a provider of consulting nutrition services to individuals and organizations. She is employed as a retail supermarket dietitian for Hannaford Brothers stores in Bangor, Maine.

Trademarks

Take It Off!

Have you ever followed a diet plan and stood in front of the scale on weigh-in day and said a silent prayer you'd actually lost weight that week? On the weeks you had less-than-stellar weigh-ins, you probably know what went wrong. It's when you kinda-sorta followed your diet that you get kinda-sorta results.

If you want quick weight-loss results, you've come to the right place. The fast-track diet program I share in this book helps you melt off stubborn weight—and drop pants sizes—over 2 months, at a pace that's both safe and motivating. You'll be eating lots of healthful, nutrient-rich foods, and you'll be rewarded with a leaner, trimmer body; more energy; and increased vitality. I've used this program with clients, and I've used it myself, so I know it works.

In this chapter, I explain how to use this weight-loss program, how to take lots of measurements before you start (and why you should), why calories count, how exercise helps you drop weight faster (and keep it off), and why you need to get plenty of rest. It's important for you to put together all the components to achieve optimum results.

What to Expect

The diet I share in this book is a healthy, balanced diet. Yet keep in mind that because you're going for accelerated results (2 months!), you're going to follow a very specific eating plan, but only for a relatively short period of time. The plan is filled with a wide variety of foods and food groups, but because it's so focused, it's not meant to be followed for a lifetime. It's designed to help the weight come off at a safe, healthy, but quick pace.

When you reach your weight-loss goal, you can gradually reintroduce some of your favorite foods and even treats to your eating plan. (Although probably not all at once—you don't want to regain all that weight!) In the meantime, you can have a reasonable treat once a week. But more on that later.

It's true that if you have more weight to lose, or are heavier or have more muscle to start with, the weight tends to come off faster than if you have less weight to lose. Everyone's body loses weight at a different rate, so if you're smaller to begin with, don't be worried or discouraged if you don't lose weight at the same pace as someone who's larger. Later in this chapter, and again in Chapter 5, we do some easy math that helps illustrate why this happens.

When you reach your goal weight, you'll need an "exit strategy" to get out of the plan without gaining back the pounds you lost. I share that later in the book, too.

Measure for Measure

Let's look at this weight-loss program as if it were a trip. You know where you want to go, right? But before you can map your journey, you have to know your current location, your starting point. That way, if you get discouraged or feel like you're not making any progress, you can look back and see how far you've come.

We're going to lock down your starting point using several methods, including taking your measurements and noting your current weight. If the thought of this makes you uncomfortable, you're not alone. I've had several personal training clients who didn't want to know how much they weighed or what their measurements were because it made them feel discouraged before they even started their diet. If this sounds like you, have someone you trust take your initial measurements, or go to a gym and ask a trainer to do it for you. It's important information to have, and later, you'll be glad to have this data.

Weighing In

First things first: weigh yourself on a good-quality scale. Note the clothes you're wearing and the time of day. I vote for weighing yourself first thing in the morning without clothes, but as long as you're consistent, it really doesn't matter. If you don't trust your scale entirely, weigh yourself three times and use the average of the three results.

TRY THIS!

Think about making Thursday or Friday your official weigh-in day. That way, if you veered a little off course over the weekend, you have a few days of on-track eating under your (hopefully smaller) belt and more chance to have undone any damage.

We're going to track your weight during the entire 2 months, on a regular basis. Just how regularly depends on you. When it comes to weigh-ins, there are two schools of thought. Most major weight-loss organizations recommend weighing yourself once a week, on the same day of the week. This way, you avoid the emotional rollercoaster that can come when the scale fluctuates a bit each day. Those fluctuations are normal based on what you're eating, your hormones, your level of rest, and a whole bunch of other factors—bodies can be finicky! Sometimes it seems that the scale randomly jumps up 1 pound and then loses 2 the next day.

Studies show, however, that daily weighing actually can help speed up your weight loss because it helps you stay on track. Some people find that this method is mentally punishing, especially if they've been working really hard, following the plan to a T, and the scale refuses to budge. If you choose daily weigh-ins, it's still a good idea to pick a day as your "official" weigh-in day to mark your progress.

We're on a tight schedule here, so I think more frequent weigh-ins are better because they can help head off problems before they get out of control. For instance, if there's something in your plan that isn't working, you don't want to lose a whole week of effort! But you decide which plan works better for you. Or split the difference and weigh on Mondays and Thursdays.

Give or Take an Inch

The scale won't be your only measure of progress. After all, the scale can be fickle. Sometimes it won't budge for a week, and sometimes it'll drop suddenly. Chances are, even if the scale didn't move, you've still lost inches.

That's why it's important to measure yourself as another way to track your progress. Get out a tape measure and be sure you're wearing clothes that aren't too bulky or too constricting (or better yet, strip down to your underwear or a bathing suit). You're going to take a whole bunch of measurements.

TRY THIS!

Did you ever notice that the ends of some tape measures are different from others? To get an accurate reading no matter what tape measure you're using, rather than measuring from the end of the tape, start measuring at 1 inch. Just be sure to subtract 1 inch from the result!

As you measure your neck, upper arm, chest, diaphragm, waist, lower abdomen, butt, thigh, knee, and calf, write down your numbers in the following table. Measure both your left and right arms and legs. These measurements change more slowly, so you're only going to measure once a week—but again, do it at the same time, wearing the same clothes.

My Measurement Chart

Measurement	Day 1	Week 1	Week 2	Week 3	Week 4
Neck					
Upper arm, left					
Upper arm, right					
Chest (men: at armpit, women: bust)					
Diaphragm (rib cage)					
Waist					
Abdomen, 6 inches below waist					
Buttocks, 9 inches below waist					
Upper thigh, left					
Upper thigh, right					
Calf, left					
Calf, right					
Upper knee, left					
Upper knee, right					

continues

My Measurement Chart   (continued)

Measurement	Week 5	Week 6	Week 7	Week 8	Total Lost
Neck					
Upper arm, left					
Upper arm, right					
Chest (men: at armpit, women: bust)					
Diaphragm (rib cage)					
Waist					
Abdomen, 6 inches below waist					
Buttocks, 9 inches below waist					
Upper thigh, left					
Upper thigh, right					
Calf, left					
Calf, right					
Upper knee, left					
Upper knee, right					

I also suggest you take pictures. I know, I know. If you're like 99 percent of my clients, you don't want anyone to see you right now wearing a swimsuit, much less take pictures of you. But don't let that stop you. If you don't want to have your picture taken in a swimsuit, try shorts and a tank top or workout clothes.

Shoot front, side, and back photos. If you have a camera with a timer, you can do this alone. I recommend taking the pictures three times: the day you begin, 1 month into the plan, and then at completion, or 8 weeks.

Later, you'll be glad you have this record of your progress. I've had many clients tell me they wish they had taken good "before" pictures. And those who do take them marvel at the change not only in their physique, but also in their facial expressions and attitudes. They often say that when they see their "before" pictures, it's as if they're looking at a different person.

Body Fat Percentage

Another measurement to consider is your body fat percentage. I'm of a mixed mind when it comes to body fat measurements. Having too much (or too little) body fat can be health hazard, so it's important information to know. However, I've seen too many clients get thrown off-course by being discouraged with their body fat results, so I often hesitate to measure it.

The number takes a while to change. It isn't always accurate; the reading result can vary based on who does the testing, how experienced the person is, how hydrated you are, and what form of measurement you're using. And often, the number comes in higher than average, which often sends people off into a frenzy of unnecessarily negative self-talk.

I've had my body fat tested by several people and through several methods. The results have ranged from 10 percent (obviously way too low) to 22 percent. One time it even came in at 33 percent (measured by an inexperienced trainer). I wasn't overweight at the time of the 33 percent measurement, and even though I knew the number was inaccurate, I felt a little deflated when I heard the result. So if you do opt to have your body fat measured, don't take the number too seriously.

However, if you want to know your body fat percentage, by all means go ahead and have it tested. Use the following table as a guide to what your numbers mean.

Body Fat Percentage Categories

	Women (% Fat)	Men (% Fat)
Essential fat	10 to 13%	2 to 5%
Athletic	14 to 20%	6 to 13%
Fit	21 to 24%	14 to 17%
Acceptable	25 to 31%	18 to 24%
Obese	32 and higher	25 and higher

Many scales now have built-in bioimpedance (BIA) measurements, and relatively inexpensive handheld devices are available that work equally well. Bioimpedance analysis devices send a very faint, imperceptible electrical charge through your body. The machine then measures the amount of resistance to the signal as it travels through the water in your body. Muscle holds more water than fat, so the more water in your body, the easier the current passes through, meaning a higher percentage of muscle to fat. The less water in your body, the more resistance to the current, meaning more fat.

TRY THIS!

The prices of body fat scales aren't that outrageous, especially if you pick them up at discount department stores. Handheld BIA devices start at around $30, while scales cost $60 and up.

Another method is to use fat calipers. I recommend you leave this method to the professionals and hire a trainer to take caliper measurements for you to ensure it's as close to accurate as possible. It's tricky to measure the right spot, and it's virtually impossible to do it yourself.

If you want the most accurate results possible, you can go to a university or a clinical setting and get an underwater hydrostatic "dunk tank" test or sit in a Bod Pod, which measures air displacement. One of the easier and more accessible options will probably work for your needs, though.

If you choose to track your body fat percentage, don't take it more than once a week because it takes a while for any real changes to register. If you choose the Bod Pod or hydrostatic options, it might make more sense to do it only at the beginning and end of your diet.

Calories Count

Ultimately, all weight loss comes down to a simple math equation:

$$\text{Calories eaten} < \text{calories burned} = \text{weight loss}$$

If you eat fewer calories than you burn, you create a calorie deficit and lose weight. Obviously, you want to create that deficit in a way that's painless and healthful so you remain energetic and feel great. But when it comes right down to it, if your goal is to lose weight, you simply have to eat fewer calories than you burn.

We're rebels about dieting, though. Many of us would rather cut out entire food groups (dairy or grains) or macronutrients (fat and carbs) than limit our energy (calorie) intake. I have some good news: with the plan in this book, you don't have to cut any food group and you don't have to count each calorie—I've already calculated that for you. However, you do have to monitor your portion sizes so you stay within a specific calorie range.

It doesn't make sense *not* to count calories (or portions). To lose 1 pound, you have to burn 3,500 calories more than you take in as fuel. You burn some of those calories just by being alive, and others are burned by exercise. (We explore this in depth starting in Chapter 5, and we also look at how to boost your calorie burn later.) So to burn 1 pound a week, you need to create a 500-calorie-a-day deficit. That's not a lot. But here's an important thing to keep in mind: it's also not hard to eat 500 (or 1,000) calories extra and undo that deficit.

When It's Okay to Cheat

Mary: "I'm so discouraged. I can't believe I didn't even lose a pound this week. I've been working so hard."

Me: "Did you follow your plan?"

Mary, taken aback: "Yes." She begins recounting what she ate that day (cereal, salad, ...).

Me: "Hmmm .... Did you have a cheat meal?"

Mary: "Well, I followed the plan perfectly last week, but I did meet friends at a restaurant Friday night and had a couple skinny margaritas. But only two. And I did have some baked tortilla chips. But I had a salad! On the weekend, my mother brought over some cupcakes for the kids. I only had one. And some pizza—my husband ordered it, and it smelled so good. I only had two small slices. Sunday I was back on track, after breakfast. We went out to eat, and I had some pancakes. But no sausage or home fries!"

This is a conversation I have all too frequently with my clients—pretty much weekly, and generally after they weigh themselves for the week.

Mary, who is trying to lose weight after having a baby a year ago, isn't alone in dieting this way—it's how most of us do it. We follow our plans during the week but then loosen up a bit on the weekend. I'm not opposed to a little treat every now and then. But when it turns into an all-out weekend off from the diet, it undoes all the effort you put in during the week.

Let's do some math: Mary is 5 foot 4 inches, weighs 165 pounds, and is 35 years old. She has a desk job and works out twice a week for 45 minutes. To maintain her weight, she needs to eat 1,805 calories a day, or 12,635 calories a week. (I get into the specifics of Mary's calorie burn and how I came up with her numbers later, in Chapter 5.) We already know that to lose 1 pound, Mary needs to create a 3,500-calorie deficit.

So say Mary eats around 1,200 calories a day, or 8,400 calories a week. She's created a caloric deficit of about 4,235—or a 1.2-pound weekly weight loss.

But then there's her diet blowout last weekend: Friday night she drank two frozen strawberry margaritas (about 300 calories total for both) and ate some salsa and chips (conservatively, 250 calories), and the salad at the restaurant came in at a whopping 700 calories—*without* dressing. On Saturday, there was the cupcake (480 calories) and two slices of pizza (250 calories each). On Sunday, she had three pancakes (450 calories).

 DANGER ZONE

Ask for nutrition info when you eat out. You'll be amazed by the calories contained in even seemingly low-calorie choices. I'm an expert on calorie counts, and I'm often stunned!

So that wiped out 2,680 calories of her deficit right there, leaving poor Mary with a deficit of only 1,555, or less than ½ pound.

If you're smaller or have less weight to lose, the margin is even tinier, so be careful when you loosen up on your diet. Even if you're grabbing a little nibble when no one's looking, the scale doesn't care. It's still counting.

That being said, if you can control your "treats," go ahead and enjoy one once a week. It's fun to make it an occasion—plan it ahead and be sure you get a chance to truly enjoy it. From a sticking-to-the-diet standpoint, it can be helpful to have your treat at night, preferably on an evening when you return to a normal schedule the next day. That way, there's a natural end point to your off-plan eating, and you're not tempted to let the "treat" mind-set slide into another treat and then another. Sunday nights are a great time to loosen up your diet a little. Many of us return to a regular schedule—which is conducive to promoting "regular" eating—on Monday morning.

Rest Up

It seems counterintuitive, but sleep is an integral part of weight loss. How can just lying in bed, snoozing, help you lose weight? It comes down to hormones. Too little sleep can throw your hormones out of whack and cause your body to hold on to that weight.

Everyone's body is a little different, but most of us need about 7 or 8 hours of sleep a night. If you're not getting that much sleep—or the sleep you're getting is poor quality—some key hormones can get out of balance. That's why we sometimes get hungry when we're overtired.

The hormones at play here are ghrelin and leptin. Ghrelin, among other things, tells you when to eat. When you're tired, you have more of it. Leptin tells you to stop eating, and when you're tired, you have less of it. When those levels get out of whack, it's no wonder it's hard to stick to a diet. Scientists are still studying the correlation between these hormones and weight. However, we know this for sure: studies show people with lower leptin levels carry more fat on their bodies.

So do what you can to get to bed on time, and practice good sleep hygiene. That doesn't mean you have to take a shower before you go to bed (although I sleep better if I do). It means you should go to sleep at a reasonable, and if possible, consistent, time each night, in a dark, cool, quiet room. Don't drink caffeinated or alcoholic beverages near bedtime, and avoid eating heavy meals a few hours before you go to bed. If sleep is an issue for you, check with your doctor to see if a sleep study is an option to figure out if there's a simple fix for the problem.

Setting Yourself Up for Success

"Fail to plan, plan to fail."

That might be a cliché, but it definitely applies in the case of weight loss. In order to succeed, you need to perform some upfront hands-on work before you start, along with some mental prep to get your head in the game.

The hands-on stuff is relatively easy—it means getting your environment in check to be as supportive of your diet as possible. Not only should you have an easy-to-follow eating plan, you also need to do as much preparation ahead of time as possible so you aren't left scrambling for something to eat at mealtime. If that happens, chances are you're going to eat something that's not part of your diet (hello, fast-food drive-thru window). Knowing there's a meal already planned and waiting for you in the fridge or freezer means you're much less apt to make that last-minute drive-thru visit. (In Chapter 9, I talk about your best options if you're forced to eat out.)

And then there's perhaps the most important element of successfully losing—and keeping off—weight: your head. In this chapter, we also look at the importance of support and how to find it in real life or online.

Putting Your Kitchen on a Diet

If you live alone, ridding your kitchen of diet obstacles is going to be a breeze. Basically, if a food isn't on your diet plan—if it's in a box, can, or bag and has a long list of ingredients, or if it contains a lot of sugar and fat—get rid of it. You can flip ahead to Chapter 3 to get an idea of the foods included in this program, which emphasizes *clean eating*. But in a nutshell, the more natural it is, the better—think fresh and frozen veggies, fruits, lean proteins, healthy fats, whole grains, and low-fat/low-sugar condiments and spices.

 DEFINITION

Clean eating is trendy these days, but it's actually how our grandparents ate. It boils down to eating unprocessed foods as close to how nature prepared them as possible, with minimal ingredients and little to no processing.

If you live with others, especially others who tend to keep tempting high-calorie foods around, try to enlist their help in keeping those foods out of your view. For instance, I have a weakness for peanut butter, which is a perfectly acceptable food, as long as you eat just a little bit of it. Keeping my peanut butter consumption to only a "little bit" sometimes can be a challenge for me. If I know it's in the cupboard, it'll call my name (especially at night if I'm tired and relaxing in front of the television) and tempt me. I've had to ask my housemate to hide the peanut butter—and even not let me know it's anywhere in the house!—so I'm not tempted to go looking for it when a craving strikes.

As you're cleaning your kitchen of off-limits food, you might hear your mother's (or in my case, my grandmother's) voice in your head admonishing you about throwing away or "wasting" perfectly good food. Ignore it! Sorry, Mom (or Nana), but if that food really *was* "perfectly good," wouldn't it be included in the diet? Yes. And if the food isn't good for you, is it good for anyone else? No. So don't feel guilty about throwing away the food. (But if it really bothers you, you always can donate it to a food pantry or leave it in the work break room.)

Why am I advocating you get rid of processed foods while you're dieting (and perhaps even after you've finished the diet)? Generally speaking, processed foods—or foods that contain lots of ingredients, especially ingredients you likely can't pronounce—don't contain the nutrients your body needs to keep it functioning optimally, especially when you're eating fewer calories in an effort to lose weight.

When you clean up your diet by eating clean—or as-close-to-natural-as-possible—foods, you get to eat more, you feel fuller longer, and your body gets more nutrition. It's a win-win-win.

Helpful Tools

You don't need a lot of expensive stuff, but a few simple items can help keep you on track. That said, it definitely helps if your fridge and freezer are large enough to accommodate the foods you'll be preparing and storing, but that shouldn't be a problem anyway, if you've done the work of clearing out the junk. (You've done that, right?)

Keeping a Food Log

Your food log can be a notebook, you can use a copy of the suggested log in this section, or you can create a document in your word-processing program. Use whatever setup feels best for you. It doesn't have to be fancy.

TRY THIS!

Many free food log websites and smartphone apps are available. Some good ones are myfitnesspal.com, fitday.com, and sparkpeople.com.

I use the notes app that came with my cell phone to record the foods I eat as I consume them, so I don't forget. At the end of the day, I email the daily memo to myself and paste it into my real log I keep on my computer. I started doing this one day when I realized I forgot to include the iced skinny coffees I enjoy on summer afternoons, which, despite being "skinny," still contain calories.

In your log, write down everything you eat, even the little tastes, nibbles, and sips of foods and calorie-containing drinks. Write down when you ate, what you ate, and how much of it you ate (or drank). You can even include your mood when you ate it.

My clients often balk at keeping a food log because they say they forget to write down stuff, it's too much work, it takes too much time, or it's a pain and they can't be bothered. My response? If they can't be bothered to keep a food log, the scale likely won't bother them much by budging.

So even if it's a pain in the butt, log your food. It'll help you find patterns in your eating that can help head off problems before they arise. And if the scale stops moving for some reason, you can go back to your food log and see what went wrong.

Remember: it's not about being perfect. It's just about having data to keep you on track toward reaching your goals!

Daily Food Log

Meal	Time Eaten	Protein	Carb	Veggie/ Fruit	Fat
Meal 1					
Meal 2					
Meal 3					
Meal 4					
Meal 5					

A Kitchen Scale

Using a food scale, you become more aware of your portion sizes. Otherwise, they have a way of getting larger without you even realizing it. (Have you ever measured out a serving size and been surprised at how small it was compared to what you used to eat?)

You don't have to use the scale every time you make meals, but it helps. I can eyeball 2 ounces of meat pretty easily, but it's easy for that 2 ounces to turn into 3 or 4 ounces over time unless I weigh regularly.

I prefer a digital scale because it allows for more precise measurements, but any kitchen scale will work. The scale doesn't have to be fancy; it simply has to be able to measure in ounces. Depending on how many extra features you want, scales cost between $8 and $100.

TRY THIS!

While we're talking portion control, you also need something to measure out those portions. Be sure you have measuring cups in ¼-, ½-, and 1-cup servings. I like to have two sets because it makes it easier when I'm preparing my meals for the week. A set of measuring spoons (teaspoon and tablespoon) is helpful, too.

Reusable Containers

I'm a big fan of reusable containers. You'll be storing both your precooked foods and your premeasured meals in them, so you'll want several, starting at about a 2-cup size and ranging up to 4 cups. You can get the inexpensive plastic ones available at the grocery or department stores, or opt for glass. The choice is yours.

Be sure to get containers that are both freezer and microwave safe. This helps cut time and mess with bulk food preparation when you can take your preprepared meals out of the freezer, defrost them in the fridge, and pop the containers into the microwave at mealtime for a quick reheat.

Zipper-lock freezer-safe baggies are good to have on hand, too.

A Food Tote

You'll likely need something in which to carry your food to and from work or school, and a collapsible food tote is perfect for this. It should be insulated to keep the food cold and safe for consumption and roomy enough to fit a couple food containers inside.

I especially like the soft-sided, insulated mini-coolers with zip-out liners. They don't take up as much room, and you can clean them easily. Don't spend a lot—good-quality totes are often available at department stores.

Plan Ahead

If you don't set aside an hour or two a couple times a week to plan and prepare your foods—especially your protein sources—in advance, it might be harder for you to stick to your diet. And that goes for just about any diet you follow—even if it's simply eating healthy foods, without regard to weight loss.

Many clients tell me they wish they were like me, with time to precook their meals. This makes me chuckle because lack of time is precisely the reason why I prepare my meals in advance. Like them, I'm time-crunched (my workday often starts before 7 A.M., and some nights I don't get home until after 8 P.M.). So I totally get that time-crunched feeling.

Clear out about an hour or so once or twice a week, a few days apart, and take some time to preplan your meals (more on this in Chapter 3) and do any necessary precooking (more on this in Chapter 4). I promise, it doesn't take a lot of time once you get a system devised.

I also try to go to the grocery store on those same days, but sometimes it doesn't work out that way.

TRY THIS!

Make 1 day a week your major cooking day, where you get the bulk of your cooking done. For most of us, this is easiest on a weekend day, when you have more time. Then, pick a weekday evening to do a smaller cooking session to prepare meals for the next couple days until the weekend rolls around again.

A bonus to this twice-weekly prep is that you usually only cook the amount of food you need, and you throw away much less food. Another bonus: grocery shopping becomes incredibly streamlined and easy, and you make fewer trips to the store, saving you money in the long run.

Getting in the Right Frame of Mind

You've already taken care of getting your environment ready for your diet. That's the easy part. The most important part is yet to come.

There's a reason many people have a hard time sticking to weight-loss plans. Even if it's the best plan in the world—and I'm pretty partial to the one in this book because it gets results, is balanced, and most importantly, is customizable to almost every palate—it won't work if their head isn't in the game. No plan will. So we're going to do some mental prep to be sure you're ready.

First, it's important to look at your *why*. Why are you embarking on this weight-loss journey? Get clear on the reasons why you're doing this. Is it to look great for a special event? Is it to fit into a certain outfit? Is it because you're interested in losing weight for health reasons? Don't skip over this part. Really take a while to think about your why. And be sure it's *your* why, not someone else's.

Losing weight is an incredibly personal journey. Not only are you changing your habits and getting out of your comfort zone, you're also changing your physical being—the body you live in 24 hours a day, 7 days a week. Making changes to it, even positive changes, can be a little daunting—as well as exciting!

When you have your reason clear, find some reminders of that reason. Okay, this might sound a little corny, but it can be a fun exercise—and great motivator!—to make a vision board to help keep you focused. Your vision board can include pictures, phrases, or anything else that reminds you of where you are headed—your why.

It's also helpful to have phrases or pictures posted where you'll regularly see them, to remind you of what you're doing and why you're doing it. Put the pictures everywhere—on the refrigerator, your computer desktop, your cell phone wallpaper, your mirror, your desk. Be sure your images and words are positive and represent something you plan to achieve. We respond much better to praise than to punishment.

For example, you could post a picture of a dress or swimsuit you plan to wear in 2 months after you've lost 20 pounds, words that have special meaning to you, or maybe a combination of the two. The reminders should resonate with you and make you feel good. Try to avoid images and words that make you feel like you're not worthy or aren't measuring up. You're fine exactly the way you are—you just want to lose a little weight, right?

Buddy Up

Studies show that people who team up with a friend or family member when following a weight-loss and exercise program tend to be more successful. That extra accountability to not only yourself but to that friend or family member can make the all difference when you're tempted to slack off a bit.

The trick, however, is to find the right buddy for you. Do you want someone who is going to work out with you? Or just someone you can check in with on a regular basis to ensure you're following your program? Do you respond best to "tough love," or do you prefer a little coddling? Think about what gets you fired up, and find someone who is capable of doing that for you. That person might not be your BFF. It might be someone else entirely—someone you might not choose to go shopping with, for example, but you know would get the job done.

It's also important that your buddy be as committed to the diet as you are. You don't want to be spending the next 2 months dragging someone along—or worse yet, have them drop out just as you're getting rolling. If you can't find your optimum person in real life, chances are you can find one online.

Some of the biggest and most active online weight-loss and fitness forums are found at sparkpeople.com, livestrong.com, myfitnesspal.com, and even bodybuilding.com. Hundreds of forums are out there—look around and find one that suits you, your personality, and your goals.

DANGER ZONE

As with all things online, do your homework, guard your privacy carefully, and be wary of those who present themselves as "experts." You never know who's actually at the other end of the keyboard.

One of my hobbies is competing in figure competitions, which is kind of like bodybuilding, except more girly. I have to follow a specific, fairly rigorous diet and workout regimen when I'm getting ready to compete, and I find it's easier to stick with my plan if I have a buddy or two I check in with regularly. Not many people—okay, pretty much no one—in my daily life understands what I go through when I'm getting ready to compete, but lots of people online do. I rely on my online workout buddies to keep me in check.

Many internet forums are free, but if you'd like to find a private site, many are available that only charge a small fee. Sometimes joining a fee-based membership site means you get a more serious, dedicated group of online buddies. No matter whether you choose free or for-pay, you'll find hundreds of other people who, like you, are following their own weight-loss and fitness journeys.

Many sites also allow you to keep an online journal of your workouts and eating program, as well as interact with others by asking and answering questions. Don't be surprised to find a great deal of support and even build lasting virtual friendships with people you meet on forums.

There's an unspoken code when it comes to successfully getting involved in forums: start by simply reading the posts, especially if they have a welcome area for new members, and then introduce yourself and treat others as you'd like to be treated. Take your time, and let people get to know you. Before long, you'll have your own virtual cheering section!

The 20 Pounds in 2 Months Plan

It's time to get to the nitty gritty of the diet that will help you lose 20 pounds in 2 months. In this chapter, we look at what foods you'll be eating over the next couple months and how you'll put them together to make meals. I designed this diet, in part, to keep your calorie intake low and still fuel your body with energy-filled carbohydrates early in the day, protein all day to keep your metabolism humming, and healthy fats later on to keep you feeling satisfied. It's also chock-full of veggies to ensure you're nourished and healthy.

As you'll see, I've classified the foods into several categories, such as protein, carbs, etc. I've arranged your daily eating plan into five meals rather than three. At each meal, you simply plug in your choices from the food categories you're supposed to eat at that time in the appropriate amount. It's really that easy!

Picky eaters, good news: if you don't like a particular food on the program, you don't have to eat it. Just pick another food choice on the list you do like. This plan is flexible and, at the same time, balanced. It's meant to work for you.

Bring on the Bulk

This plan allows you to eat meals that give you plenty of "bulk" to keep your tummy happy—and much of that bulk comes from veggies chock full of fiber. It's important to remember that it takes about 20 minutes after you start eating for your brain to say, "I'm full!" so meals that take a little longer to eat will be more satisfying. Think of veggies as your go-to food for feeling full, so load up a big plate (or bowl) full of them.

The veggies included in this program will definitely fill you up. And your body will love what all those nutrient-dense veggies do for it, infusing it with vitamins and minerals. Plenty of yummy condiments you can use to jazz up those veggies and other meals to keep your taste buds happy are included in the program.

Designing Your Meals

You'll be eating every 3 or 4 hours with this program. That way, you'll always have a meal to look forward to, and your metabolism will keep chugging along as your body is continually busy digesting food. It also will keep your blood sugar stable, which studies show is important not only for weight loss but general health.

Here's how you'll design your meals (the food choices you'll plug into the meal plan are coming right up):

> **Meal 1:** Protein, carb, fruit (vegetable optional)
>
> **Meal 2:** Protein, carb, fruit (vegetable optional)
>
> **Meal 3:** Protein, carb, vegetable (for those following Plan D, add 1 serving of good fat and 1 fruit)
>
> **Meal 4:** Protein, vegetable, good fat
>
> **Meal 5:** Protein, vegetable, good fat

If you're not used to eating five times a day, you might go through an adjustment period as your body adapts to the more regular feedings. In fact, the first day or two, you might be tempted to skip a meal because you feel full. Please try to eat all the meals; otherwise, later in the week you likely will end up with a growling, hungry stomach and feel ready to dive headfirst into something that's not going to help you get to your goal weight!

TRY THIS!

If, after a few days following this plan, you find that eating five times a day makes you continually think about food, or the more-frequent meals just don't work with your schedule, you can cut the number of meals back to four. Just be sure to fold the omitted foods into one or two of your other meals (preferably earlier in the day) by bumping up the portion sizes slightly.

I also specifically call each of these "feedings" a meal for a reason—if I called any of the meals "snacks," chances are (especially if you're anything like me!) you'd start thinking about something super sugary/salty/high-calorie, and that's definitely not on the plan. So for now, let's get rid of the word snack from your vocabulary. Your meals are meals.

Making Smart Food Choices

This eating plan is all about nutrient density and includes foods that give you the most nutrition bang for your calorie buck. The foods are "clean"—that is, not processed—and help keep you feeling energetic, healthy, and nourished as you reduce your calories for a safe, optimum level of weight loss. As a bonus, you'll experience reduced cravings, improved energy, and better results with these smart choices. And when you monitor not only your portion sizes, but also your food choices, your results will skyrocket!

DANGER ZONE

Avoid artificial sweeteners whenever possible because, among other things, they actually can *escalate* cravings.

It's important to note that you should eat from a wide variety of food choices within each section to ensure you get a broad range of nutrients, vitamins, and minerals. You won't have to count calories in this plan, but depending on what you choose within each section, your daily caloric intake may vary a bit.

I've done most of the figuring for you, but because we're all different, with our own unique metabolism, activity level, and more, the more specific we can get, the better. In Chapter 5, I point you to some handy gadgets to help you more precisely track your calorie intake so you can tweak this plan to your needs. But for now, this will definitely get you started.

The following figures are based on caloric need estimates of average Americans from the Dietary Guidelines for Americans, 2010, U.S. Department of Agriculture, U.S. Department of Health and Human Services. The USDA estimated about how many calories the average American (defined as a 5-foot, 10-inch-tall man weighing 154 pounds and a 5-foot, 4-inch-tall woman weighing 126 pounds) needs to maintain his or her weight.

We'll get into the math that's involved with weight loss later, but know this: to lose at least 2 pounds a week (which will put you on the fast track), you have to create a 1,000-calorie deficit every day. To do that, check out which plan you should follow based on your activity level.

Which Plan Is for You?

Gender	Sedentary	Moderately Active	Active
Female	Plan A	Plan A	Plan B
Male	Plan B	Plan C	Plan D

A sedentary physical activity level includes the light activity that normally occurs in regular everyday life—walking around the house, showering, doing chores, etc.

Moderately active includes the normal everyday activities, plus the equivalent of walking about 1½ to 3 miles a day at 3 or 4 miles an hour.

Active refers to the normal activities plus walking so that you're racking up more than 3 miles a day.

The calorie allotment per plan is as follows:

- Plan A contains an estimated 1,200 calories, depending on the food choices you make within the plan.
- Plan B contains an estimated 1,500 calories.
- Plan C comes in at around 2,000 calories.
- Plan D contains about 2,250 calories.

Note this is a very broad estimate of how many calories you should eat to lose weight, based on figures from the U.S. government's 2010 dietary guidelines. Later, in Chapter 5, we fine-tune these figures to be more reflective of your specific needs based on your age, activity level, weight, height, and gender.

Choose Your Food

The following sections list the food options you can plug into your plan, and how much of each you get to eat to stay on-plan, depending on how many calories you need to achieve your goal based on gender, age, and activity level.

Protein

Getting adequate protein helps keep your blood sugar stable and your cravings at bay. When you're dieting, eating protein also helps ensure you're preserving muscle as the weight comes off.

Protein

Food	Plan A	Plan B	Plan C	Plan D
Chicken breast	2 oz.	3 oz.	5 oz.	5 oz.
Cottage cheese (1% fat)	½ cup	¾ cup	1 cup	1 cup
Eggs	4 egg whites	1 egg plus 4 egg whites	1 egg plus 4 egg whites	1 egg plus 4 egg whites
Extra-lean ground turkey	2 oz.	3 oz.	5 oz.	5 oz.
Greek yogurt (fat-free, plain)	½ cup	¾ cup	1 cup	1 cup
Haddock, cod, or other whitefish, broiled or grilled	3 oz.	5 oz.	6 oz.	6 oz.
Lean beef or steak	2 oz.	3 oz.	5 oz.	5 oz.
Lobster	3 oz.	4 oz.	5 oz.	5 oz.
Salmon	2.5 oz.	5 oz.	6 oz.	6 oz.
Scallops	3 oz.	4 oz.	5 oz.	5 oz.
Shrimp	3 oz.	4 oz.	5 oz.	5 oz.
Tilapia	3 oz.	5 oz.	6 oz.	6 oz.
Tuna (packed in water)	3 oz.	3 oz.	5 oz.	5 oz.
Turkey breast	2 oz.	3 oz.	5 oz.	5 oz.
Whey protein (2 times a day if using)	1 scoop or 18 grams protein	1 scoop or 18 grams protein	1 scoop or 18 grams protein	1½ scoops or 30 grams protein

TRY THIS!

Always opt for healthy preparation methods like broiling and grilling. Stay away from fried, battered, or baked-in-butter-and-sprinkled-in-Ritz-crackers dishes!

Carbohydrates (Starches)

Don't skimp on the starchy carbs—just be sure to watch your portion sizes, as the calories add up quickly. You'll fuel up with carbs early in the day to give you valuable energy.

Carbs

Food	Plan A	Plan B	Plan C	Plan D
Barley, cooked	½ cup	¾ cup	1 cup	1 cup
Bread, 100% whole grain	1 slice	1 slice	2 slices	2 slices
Brown rice, cooked	½ cup	¾ cup	1 cup	1 cup
Cooked dried beans	½ cup	¾ cup	1 cup	1 cup
Couscous, cooked	½ cup	¾ cup	1 cup	1 cup
Lentils, cooked	½ cup	¾ cup	1 cup	1 cup
Oat bran cereal	⅓ cup	½ cup	¾ cup	¾ cup
Old-fashioned (not instant) oatmeal, unprepared	¼ cup	½ cup	¾ cup	¾ cup
Pumpkin, canned	¾ cup	1 cup	1½ cups	1½ cups

continues

Carbs (continued)

Food	Plan A	Plan B	Plan C	Plan D
Quinoa, cooked	½ cup	¾ cup	1 cup	1 cup
Shredded wheat cereal	¾ cup	1 cup	1 cup	1½ cups
Spaghetti squash, cooked	2 cups	3 cups	4 cups	4 cups
Sweet potatoes	½ cup	¾ cup	1 cup	1 cup
White and red potatoes	½ cup	¾ cup	1 cup	1 cup
Wrap, low-carb whole grain (less than 100 calories each)	1 wrap	1 wrap	2 wraps	2 wraps

Fruits and Vegetables

All fresh fruits—no sweeteners—are acceptable. Frozen fruits are also permitted as long as they're not frozen in syrup. Canned foods are okay as long as they're canned in juice or water.

A serving size equals 1 medium piece of fruit or ½ cup.

Fruits

Food	Plan A	Plan B	Plan C	Plan D
Fruit	2 servings	2 servings	2 servings	3 servings

All nonstarchy vegetables—such as green beans, broccoli, asparagus, cauliflower, spinach, etc.—are acceptable.

If you aren't used to eating many vegetables, be sure to gradually increase the amount you're eating, as large amounts can cause digestive distress if suddenly introduced to your diet.

TRY THIS!

Fruits and vegetables are carbohydrates—and so are the starchy carbohydrates listed in this plan. Why are they classified separately? Among other reasons: nutrient density (the good stuff they contain per calorie), fiber, and sugar content. Starchy carbs contain three or more sugars; fruits and vegetables contain one or two forms of sugar.

Aim for 1 or more cups per meal. As you'll note in the sample daily meal plans at the end of this chapter, 2 cups veggies are included in a couple meals.

Lettuce, mushrooms, celery, onions, bell peppers, and cucumbers are "free," within reason. If you eat more than 3 cups a day, include them as a vegetable serving.

Good Fats

Don't avoid fats when you're dieting. Some fats are actually beneficial for you and keep you feeling fuller longer. They also keep your skin and hair looking great.

Good Fats

Food	Plan A	Plan B	Plan C	Plan D
Almonds and other nuts	½ oz.	½ oz.	½ oz.	½ oz.
Avocado, sliced	½ cup	½ cup	¾ cup	1½ cups
Black olives, large, pitted	12 olives	12 olives	20 olives	20 olives
Canola oil	1 TB.	1 TB.	1½ TB.	1½ TB.
Coconut oil	1 TB.	1 TB.	1½ TB.	1½ TB.
Flax oil	1 TB.	1 TB.	1½ TB.	1½ TB.
Olive oil	1 TB.	1 TB.	1½ TB.	1½ TB.
Tahini paste	1 TB.	1 TB.	1½ TB.	1½ TB.

Other Ingredients

Beyond the foundation of the diet—protein, carbs, and fats—your body also needs other food groups for health. Your taste buds will appreciate them, too!

Dairy products Aim for 1 or 2 nonfat (or if using cottage cheese, low-fat, as nonfat contains more sodium) servings per day.

Condiments Use at will: mustard, ketchup, fat-free/low-sugar/noncreamy salad dressings, vinegar, spice blends, salsa, flavor extracts.

Beverages Water. Try to drink ½ to 1 gallon water a day. If you haven't been drinking this much and are exercising regularly, gradually increase your water each week slowly. Try to limit other, calorie-free beverages—such as coffee and tea—to a couple servings per day.

Multivitamins Take a good-quality multivitamin and/or fish oil supplement, *as recommended by your physician or pharmacist.*

A Sample Day's Diet

Here's an idea of how to put the eating plan together. Again, your choices might vary based on your food preference, what's in the cupboard, or even your schedule.

Plan A:

> **Meal 1:** 4 scrambled egg whites, ¾ cup shredded wheat cereal with a splash of skim milk, ½ cup orange slices, 1 cup coffee

> **Meal 2:** ½ cup plain nonfat Greek yogurt with ¼ cup dry oatmeal stirred in, along with ½ cup berries

> **Meal 3:** 2 ounces grilled turkey breast, ½ cup sweet potato, 2 cups veggies

Meal 4: $\frac{1}{2}$ cup low-fat cottage cheese with $\frac{1}{2}$ ounce walnuts and 1 cup baby carrots, unlimited iced green tea

Meal 5: 2 ounces chicken breast sautéed with 2 cups frozen, chopped spinach in 1 tablespoon olive oil

Plan B:

Meal 1: 4 egg whites and 1 whole egg, scrambled; 1 cup shredded wheat cereal with a splash of skim milk; $\frac{1}{2}$ cup orange slices; 1 cup coffee

Meal 2: $\frac{3}{4}$ cup plain nonfat Greek yogurt with $\frac{1}{2}$ cup dry oatmeal stirred in, along with $\frac{1}{2}$ cup berries

Meal 3: 3 ounces grilled turkey breast, $\frac{1}{2}$ cup sweet potato, 2 cups veggies

Meal 4: $\frac{3}{4}$ cup low-fat cottage cheese with $\frac{1}{2}$ ounce walnuts and 1 cup baby carrots, unlimited iced green tea

Meal 5: 3 ounces chicken breast sautéed with 2 cups frozen, chopped spinach in 1 tablespoon olive oil

Plan C:

Meal 1: 4 egg whites and 1 whole egg, scrambled; 1 cup shredded wheat cereal with a splash of skim milk; $\frac{1}{2}$ cup orange slices; 1 cup coffee

Meal 2: 1 cup plain nonfat Greek yogurt with $\frac{3}{4}$ cup dry oatmeal stirred in, along with $\frac{1}{2}$ cup berries

Meal 3: 5 ounces grilled chicken breast, 1 cup sweet potato, 2 cups veggies

Meal 4: 1 cup low-fat cottage cheese with $\frac{1}{4}$ ounce walnuts and 1 cup baby carrots, unlimited iced green tea

Meal 5: 5 ounces chicken breast sautéed with 2 cups frozen, chopped spinach in 1 tablespoon olive oil

Plan D:

Meal 1: 4 egg whites and 1 whole egg, scrambled; 1 cup shredded wheat cereal with a splash of skim milk; ½ cup orange slices; 1 cup coffee

Meal 2: 1 cup plain nonfat Greek yogurt with ¼ cup dry oatmeal stirred in, along with ½ cup berries

Meal 3: 5 ounces grilled chicken breast, 1 cup sweet potato, 2 cups veggies sautéed in 1½ tablespoons olive oil, 1 apple

Meal 4: 1 cup low-fat cottage cheese with ½ ounce walnuts and 1 cup baby carrots, unlimited iced green tea

Meal 5: 5 ounces chicken breast sautéed with 2 cups frozen, chopped spinach in 1½ tablespoons olive oil

Putting It All Together

You've mapped your journey, gathered your tools, assembled your support crew, and put on your game face. Now it's time to put all your planning to work.

In this chapter, I explain how to get all your food put together for an entire week so you don't run into any last-minute stumbling blocks. We figure out your key meals, learn smart grocery shopping, set up a meal assembly line so you can get as much of the meal prep done as possible, and get your meals all set for the week—or maybe even longer, with the help of your freezer.

Meal planning and preparation is the most-discussed topic among my training clients, and many people struggle with it. It makes sense: when you're driving home from work with a growling stomach and feeling tired from the day, the last thing you want to do is go home and figure out what to cook for supper. It's tempting to make a detour through the drive-thru or call for a pizza delivery and vow to start afresh with your diet in the morning.

A couple hours of upfront work (at the most, and it will take less time than that once you get your own system devised) is a small price to pay for the quality-of-life improvement of having food waiting for you at home. Not only will you no longer have to stress about what's for dinner, but you'll also save money by avoiding those last-minute food purchases. You'll also feel better by avoiding fat-laden, sodium-heavy, and sugary foods!

If you're struggling with finding the time, think back to the "why" you established in Chapter 2 for losing the weight, and get a little selfish. Look at one of the reminders you have posted nearby. (You didn't skip that step, did you?) Guard your time and make it happen!

Updating Your Go-To Meals

Having a few meals you enjoy and that are easy to prepare makes cooking so much easier. Chances are you already have several "go-to" meals that are your favorites or standards: your muffin and coffee for breakfast, your sandwich/salad for lunch, or your ritual Friday night pizza. All you're going to do here is exchange those choices for some more diet-friendly ones.

When you swap out your current meals for new, healthier ones, it's important to eat a variety of foods to ensure you're getting all the nutrients you need. Eating chicken and broccoli five times a day might help you lose weight, but it certainly won't make you, or your body, happy long-term.

But you don't want to make your food choices too wide either, for a couple reasons. If you're frugal and no one else in your household is following your plan, you want to be sure you actually eat all the food you're preparing to avoid having to throw a bunch of food away.

And then there's what I call the buffet effect. If you're like many people, when you stand in front of a buffet of food, you may feel compelled to eat until you're stuffed. Or when you've prepared a special recipe, you might eat more of it than you would a normal meal. Studies have shown that the bigger the variety of foods we're presented with, the more calories we eat. That's why it's a good idea to stick with your go-to meals, so you don't splurge when presented with constantly changing new choices.

Sit down with the food plan from Chapter 3 and come up with a list of possible meals you can enjoy over the next week. In my experience, the simpler the meals, the better—it's less fuss and trouble to make them, and when you're dieting, the less time you have to spend thinking about food, the better.

Now figure out a few combinations for each meal before you get started. I find it's easiest to begin with the protein choice and add to that. In Chapter 3, I outlined a sample day's meal plan. Let's take that a step further and come up with a few more.

Here are some possibilities for meals 1 and 2:

> Eggs, oatmeal, and ½ orange
>
> Greek yogurt, berries, and whole-wheat toast
>
> A protein shake smoothie with 1 scoop protein powder, ¼ cup oatmeal, and ½ banana
>
> Cottage cheese with pineapple and a sprinkling of oat-based, low-fat granola

Some lunch (meal 3) choices:

> Veggie and greens salad with tuna and cannellini beans
>
> Whole-grain wrap with turkey, spinach, and veggies
>
> Chicken with sweet potato and broccoli

Choices for meals 4 and 5:

> Chicken or fish with veggies sautéed in coconut or olive oil
>
> A chocolate protein shake with 1 tablespoon peanut butter
>
> Beef and broccoli stir-fry in coconut or olive oil

Again, these are just examples, so feel free to choose foods you enjoy. And as you're customizing your menu, think about ways to add healthy, no- or low-calorie flavors to your dishes. Try lemon juice with fish, a spice rub, balsamic vinegar, or maybe even some buffalo wing sauce. Be creative!

When you have your meals planned, it's time to go shopping.

At the Grocery Store

You've probably heard the advice, and it's true: never go grocery shopping when you're hungry. And always go armed with a list, preferably arranged according to the layout of the store to avoid detours into danger zones (the chip aisle, the ice-cream freezer, the bakery—the areas that most test your willpower). This is going to be your fastest, easiest shopping experience ever!

In the produce section, check out the prepared fresh veggies. A variety of slaws—coleslaw (shredded cabbage), broccoli slaw (shredded cabbage, broccoli, and carrots), and rainbow slaw (shredded cabbage, broccoli, cauliflower, and carrots)—are available that you can quickly toss with other meals to add bulk with minimal calories. They're also great tossed with a light salad dressing or balsamic vinegar.

In the bakery area, if bread is on your list, carefully review the ingredients list to be sure it's whole grain—the marketing on the wrapper itself can be deceiving. Check that the first ingredient is "whole-wheat flour" or "100 percent whole wheat." Obviously, steer clear of the cakes, donuts, and cookies!

When it comes to the freezer veggies, I tend to buy bags of frozen organic vegetables and berries: green beans, broccoli, spinach, and more. They're convenient, don't spoil, and depending on the season, contain nearly the same nutrient quality as fresh vegetables and fruits.

TRY THIS!

Whenever possible, eat fresh vegetables and fruits in season, preferably from local farms. When you buy local, there's less lag time between when the produce was picked at the farm to when it arrives on your table, ensuring a high nutrient value. If that's not possible, frozen veggies are a good alternative. They also are picked at the peak of freshness and immediately frozen, with minimal nutrient loss. Some canned vegetables—like pumpkin and tomatoes—are comparable to or better than fresh varieties, nutrition-wise.

Reading labels is key, and not just when it comes to ingredients. When you're choosing meats and other proteins, always check the sell-by/use-by date to be sure it's fresh. This is especially important if you're cooking in bulk.

When you're choosing salad dressing and condiments, examine the labels to be sure they aren't loaded with ingredients you can't identify and that they don't contain excess fat, sugar, or calories. Better yet, make your own dressings by mixing balsamic vinegar, healthy oils (like flax), and spices!

In the spice aisle, check out some of the spice blends, which can help add zip to vegetables or grilled meats.

When choosing yogurt, oatmeal, or other foods that often come already flavored (and usually with a hefty dose of sugar thrown in for added taste), opt for plain. You easily can flavor these foods yourself using lower-calorie, lower-sugar options.

Cooking in Bulk

Now that you have a kitchen full of fresh, healthful food, it's time to get cooking—in bulk! Bulk cooking is actually pretty easy. It's sort of like cooking a big family meal, except you're not going to sit down to eat it when it's done. Instead, you're going to pack it all up like leftovers to enjoy later.

Many of our grandmothers used to cook triple batches of foods and store them for later. In fact, if you check out some frugal cooking websites online, you'll see bulk cooking is a popular money-saving tactic in use today. You're doing the same thing, except you're saving calories and banking your time. The process itself is simple: just figure out how many servings of which food you're going to need and start cooking.

TRY THIS!

I like to listen to music or podcasts when I do my bulk cooking to make it seem less like a chore and more like an occasion.

Low and Slow Cooking

If you have a slow cooker—and if you don't, consider buying one—you can get a jump on meal prep early in the day you plan on bulk cooking. Scores of simple, healthy slow cooker recipes are available in cookbooks and online, but it's easy to create your own. The great thing about slow cooker cooking is that it's nearly foolproof as long as you choose tasty ingredients.

To devise your own recipe, choose a protein (chicken breasts and lean beef are both great options, and 1 pound yields 3 to 8 meals, depending on your portion sizes) and cut it into cubes. Next, pick a low-fat sauce (for chicken, salsa or buffalo wing sauce are yummy choices; for beef, how about low-sodium/low-sugar teriyaki sauce?).

Give the slow cooker crock a quick spray with nonstick cooking spray. Layer some sauce in the bottom of the slow cooker, add your protein, and then add just enough sauce to cover the protein. Cook, stirring once or twice, on medium for 3 or 4 hours or until done. When the meat falls apart as you cut it, it's done!

When it's almost time for the food in the slow cooker to be done, I begin to prepare the rest of the foods that will see me through the week.

Veggie Prep

Next I chop some onions and peppers, put them in a preheated nonstick skillet with a little bit of water or cooking spray, and "fry" them. Then I add 1 pound ground turkey or chicken breast (again, 6 to 8 servings) to brown.

In a separate pan, I sauté some other veggies in advance— remember, they're free, calorie-wise, and can be used for flavor and to add some extra bulk your meals. I generally sauté onions, mushrooms, and peppers, but you can add summer squash, zucchini, carrots, spinach, or whatever happens to be in your fridge at the time. I make a lot, store them in a container, and add them to other meals as I crave them.

While all that's going on, I often put a sweet potato or two in the microwave to cook. If you prefer, you can put a pot of brown rice on the stove to simmer.

TRY THIS!

There are three tricks to perfectly steamed rice. Use a large saucepan with a tight-fitting lid to allow more even disbursement of heat. And simmer the rice on your stove's lowest-heat "simmer" burner. Also, be sure to use the proper ratio of water to rice: for 1 cup rice, use 2½ cups water. To cook, bring the rice and water to a boil, reduce heat to low, and simmer, covered, for about 40 to 45 minutes or until most of the liquid has been absorbed. Let stand for 5 minutes, fluff with a fork, and serve.

Some Assembly Required

When your various ingredients are finished cooking, it's time to start assembling your meals. This is when you need to gather your tools: your scale, measuring cups, reusable food containers, and freezer-friendly zipper-lock bags.

You have two choices—you can either portion out all your foods separately, or you can create one-dish meals. I'm a big fan of one-dish meals because they're easy, take up less room in the refrigerator and freezer, and require less thinking on my part during the busy week ahead.

To make one-dish meals, set your reusable container on the food scale, zero out the weight of the container, and add the appropriate amount of protein. Then, if the meal you're preparing contains a starch, measure and add that, followed by your veggies. Cover the container, label it, and date it. I like to place a piece of plain cellophane tape on the lid and write on it with a permanent marker. The tape is easy to remove later. Repeat for each meal, and voilà! You're done!

Then place the containers for the next couple days in the fridge. Allow the other containers to cool in the refrigerator, and place them in the freezer for use later in the week.

If you build up a stockpile of frozen premade meals, you can cut back a bit on the precooking. Plus, when you make a fresh meal, make a double or triple batch so you freeze the leftovers for eating later.

 TRY THIS!

For best results, freeze the food at its peak of quality, soon after it has been cooked. Don't wait a couple days and decide to freeze it at the last minute because you're afraid it might spoil. You'll lose valuable nutrients.

If you're not a fan of one-dish meals or would prefer to store your foods separately, simply weigh your protein choices and put them into reusable containers or zipper-lock freezer bags. If you plan on freezing your proteins, be sure the container isn't too big or else air could get trapped inside, resulting in a less-than-tasty freezer-burned meal.

Enjoying the Fruits of Your Labor

When you've completed the meal preparation, stand back and enjoy the view of your now-full fridge. Pretty, isn't it? Now your only job for meal prep is to be sure each night that your food is ready to roll for the next day. For frozen foods, this might mean moving the container from the freezer to the fridge so it has a chance to thaw.

Here's what my evening ritual looks like: each night after I finish eating my dinner, I make sure my meals for the next day are ready—this takes maybe 5 minutes, tops. I'm a morning procrastinator, so if I plan on having Greek yogurt for breakfast, I stir in my berries the night before so the yogurt has a chance to pick up that extra flavor as it sits overnight. Sometimes, if I know I'm going to be especially rushed in the morning and eggs are on my menu, I even cook the eggs the night before. The next morning, all I have to do is grab my breakfast out of the fridge, reheat it if necessary, and eat. I put my other meals for the day into my mini cooler, and I'm ready to go!

It's not rocket science, so try not to overthink the meal prep. The most important thing is to make the time to do it. And then, the more often you precook, the easier it gets and the less time it takes.

A Week of Meals

Your portion sizes will correspond with the number of calories you're allotted in the specific diet plan you're following (A, B, C, or D). The meals all start with a protein choice, with an added starch during the first three meals to fuel you through the day. Every meal includes a fruit or vegetable option.

Day 1:

> **Meal 1:** Plain Greek yogurt with dry oatmeal and blueberries stirred in, sweetened with stevia
>
> **Meal 2:** Protein shake with banana and shredded wheat cereal
>
> **Meal 3:** Large veggie salad with balsamic vinegar sprinkled with black beans and grilled chicken
>
> **Meal 4:** Cottage cheese with baby carrots and walnuts
>
> **Meal 5:** Haddock with vegetables (onions, peppers, broccoli, and carrots) sautéed in coconut oil

Day 2:

> **Meal 1:** Egg whites scrambled with salsa and spinach, whole-wheat toast, orange slices
>
> **Meal 2:** Plain Greek yogurt with dry oatmeal and blueberries stirred in, sweetened with stevia
>
> **Meal 3:** Turkey breast and veggies in a whole-grain wrap with baby carrots on the side
>
> **Meal 4:** Chocolate protein shake with peanut butter
>
> **Meal 5:** Chicken and veggies stir-fried in olive oil

Day 3:

> **Meal 1:** Whole-wheat toast with cottage cheese and pineapple
>
> **Meal 2:** Protein shake with oatmeal and 1 orange
>
> **Meal 3:** Large veggie salad with balsamic vinegar sprinkled with black beans and grilled chicken
>
> **Meal 4:** Chicken and green beans
>
> **Meal 5:** Chocolate protein shake with peanut butter and 1 tablespoon cocoa powder

Day 4:

> **Meal 1:** Egg whites scrambled with salsa and spinach, slice of whole-wheat toast, $\frac{1}{2}$ banana for those following plans A and B and 1 whole banana for those following plans C and D
>
> **Meal 2:** Whole-wheat toast with cottage cheese and pineapple
>
> **Meal 3:** Turkey breast with sweet potato and broccoli and green beans, drizzled with balsamic vinegar
>
> **Meal 4:** Haddock with rainbow slaw and green beans sautéed in coconut oil
>
> **Meal 5:** Protein shake with almonds

Day 5:

> **Meal 1:** Plain nonfat Greek yogurt with dry oatmeal and blueberries stirred in, sweetened with stevia
>
> **Meal 2:** Protein shake with banana and shredded wheat cereal
>
> **Meal 3:** Chicken, brown rice, broccoli
>
> **Meal 4:** Grilled shrimp with a large vegetable salad drizzled with a flax-balsamic vinaigrette
>
> **Meal 5:** Cottage cheese, almonds, baby carrots

Day 6:

> **Meal 1:** Egg whites scrambled with salsa and spinach, whole-wheat toast, 1 orange
>
> **Meal 2:** Toasted whole-grain wrap smothered in cottage cheese, mushrooms, spinach, and onions; banana

TRY THIS!

Meal 2's wrap is fantastic warm. After you've assembled the wrap, bake it in a 350°F oven for 5 to 8 minutes.

Meal 3: Chicken, brown rice, green beans

Meal 4: Protein shake with berries and almonds

Meal 5: Haddock, broccoli with flax oil and vinegar as dressing

Day 7:

Meal 1: Plain Greek yogurt with dry oatmeal and blueberries stirred in, sweetened with stevia

Meal 2: Protein shake with banana and shredded wheat cereal

Meal 3: Large veggie salad with chicken and black beans, with a flax-balsamic vinaigrette

Meal 4: Shrimp sautéed in coconut oil with broccoli

Meal 5: Haddock with rainbow slaw and green beans sautéed in coconut oil

Boosting Your Burn

With weight loss, the bottom line is always the same: you have to burn more calories than you take in. When that happens, your body begins using as fuel what it used to store as fat. The more you move over the course of a day, the more calories you burn, and as a result, the more weight you lose. It's that simple.

So it makes sense that if you want faster weight-loss results, you need to increase how much you move. (There are other reasons to increase your activity level, but I get into those later.) Because you're on a fast-track to weight loss here, increasing your calorie burn is an important part of the weight-loss equation.

How Your Body Burns Calories

Your body burns calories in a number of different ways. The most basic is by simply being alive and powering your organs. That's your basal metabolic rate, or BMR. You also burn calories as you go about the business of living your life (walking from room to room, brushing your teeth, making and cooking meals, etc.). And on top of that, you burn calories while exercising and even *after* exercising, which we explore in Chapter 6.

Your BMR is pretty much static, so we're going to look at ways to boost how many calories you burn through the means most easily controlled: how much you move over the course of the day and also your exercise-related calories. We're going to look at increasing your *nonexercise activity thermogenesis* (*NEAT*). That's a fancy term for how many calories you burn while you're living your life. Just sitting around doesn't generate much NEAT. Gardening or playing with your kids does.

 DEFINITION

> **Nonexercise activity thermogenesis (NEAT)** is the amount of energy you burn over the course of the day at work, at home, and at play, separate from exercise. Experts believe NEAT calories play a large role in overall weight regulation, accounting for as many as 50 percent of calories you use. The more you move, the more you burn!

Then, of course, there's intentional calorie burning, or exercise. When it comes to weight loss, we can break exercise into two categories: resistance (strength) training and cardiovascular activities (what we used to call aerobics), each of which makes a unique contribution to weight loss. (I outline ways to optimize both kinds of workouts for fat-burning in the next two chapters.)

Calculating Your Burn

So how much energy—that is, how many calories—do you burn in a day? We can get a ballpark figure using some basic math.

The first thing we need to do is use something called the Harris-Benedict equation for calculating your BMR. Remember, your BMR is the number of calories you'd burn a day if you don't do anything. The formula used to come up with this calculation might look a little scary—but never fear! If I can figure this out, so can you. Let's look at it together.

Here's the equation for women:

> BMR = 655 + (4.35 × weight in pounds) + (4.7 × height in inches) − (4.7 × age in years)

Here's the equation for men:

> BMR = 66 + (6.23 × weight in pounds) + (12.7 × height in inches) − (6.8 × age in years)

Now let's do the calculations. Remember Mary from Chapter 1? She's 35 years old, stands 5 feet, 4 inches tall, and weighs 165 pounds. Let's plug Mary's numbers into the calculation:

> BMR = 655 + (4.35 × 165) + (4.7 × 64) − (4.7 × 35)

If you remember from math class, you always do the calculations inside the parentheses first. Doing that, the equation now looks like this (I've rounded numbers slightly where appropriate):

> BMR = 655 + 718 + 301 − 165
>
> BMR = 1,509

That means that without even getting up to move, Mary burns 1,509 calories every day. Not too shabby!

Let's meet Bob, who stands 5 feet, 11 inches tall, and weighs 230 pounds. Bob is 38 years old. Here's his BMR:

> BMR = 66 + (6.23 × 230) + (12.7 × 71) − (6.8 × 38)
>
> BMR = 66 + 1,433 + 902 − 258
>
> BMR = 2,143

So Bob burns 2,143 calories a day if he doesn't get out of bed.

The next thing we need to do is calculate Mary's and Bob's daily caloric burn—their *total daily energy expenditure* (*TDEE*), which includes their BMR, NEAT calories, and any calories they might burn exercising.

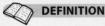

> Your **total daily energy expenditure (TDEE)** is the number of calories your body burns over the course of a day. To maintain your weight, you must create a balance between calorie consumption and TDEE. To lose 1 pound weight per week, you have to eat 500 calories per day less than you burn; to lose 2 pounds per week, you have to increase that deficit to 1,000 calories a day.

The less active you are, the fewer "extra" calories you need to fuel your daily activities. When you're trying to lose weight, those "extra" calories make the difference between a happy weigh-in day and a frustrating one.

Sedentary (little to no exercise): calories = BMR × 1.2

Lightly active (light exercise/sports 1 to 3 days a week): calories = BMR × 1.375

Moderately active (moderate exercise/sports 3 to 5 days a week): calories = BMR × 1.55

Very active (hard exercise/sports 6 or 7 days a week): calories = BMR × 1.725

Extra active (very hard exercise/sports and physical job or twice-a-day training): calories = BMR × 1.9

A word of warning: we all tend to overestimate our activity level, just as we all tend to underestimate how many calories we eat. Even I do it, and I'm a trained professional. When I first calculated my calorie burn, I thought for sure I fell into the "extra active" category. I mean, I'm a personal trainer. I lift weights not only when I work out but also for other people all day when I'm demonstrating exercises. Plus, I teach exercise classes and do cardio a few times a week. Turns out, I'm not in the extra active group. I'm in the "very active" group.

So let's say Mary has a sedentary job. She sits at a desk most of the day, but she does go for a 30-minute walk a few nights a week with her husband—Bob!—when the weather is nice. (Despite the walks, I'm going to say Mary is sedentary, the first group. A few leisurely strolls a week that don't cause her to break a sweat don't constitute "exercise.") Bob also has a sedentary job, and his only activities are the evening strolls with Mary.

To find their TDEEs, we simply multiply their BMRs by their activity levels, which we're estimating at 1.2—sedentary with little to no exercise:

> Mary: 1,509 × 1.2 = 1,811 calories a day
>
> Bob: 2,143 × 1.2 = 2,572 calories a day

If Mary follows the eating plan to a T but doesn't change her activity at all, she's on track to lose about 1.2 pounds a week. (Remember, to lose 1 pound a week, you need to create a 3,500-calorie deficit, or 500 calories a day. To lose 2 pounds a week, you need to boost that deficit to 1,000 calories a day.)

Now, let's say we get her to the gym 4 or 5 days a week, and she makes it a point to be more active at work when she can—standing more, taking some short walks at lunchtime or on breaks. In that case, we can boost her to the "moderately active" group, making her on track to lose 2.25 pounds a week (that's her weight, 165, multiplied by 1.55). In the course of a week, the 1-pound difference might not seem like much, but in 8 weeks, that difference is impressive. Without changing her activity, she would lose 9.6 pounds. By changing her activity, her weight loss jumps to 18.6 pounds.

That extra weight loss makes those workouts and daily movement tweaks a little more appealing, doesn't it?

Gadgets to Get You Going

If you're a gadget freak (like me!), some fun products can help you track how much you move, how many steps you take, and how many NEAT calories you burn over the course of a day.

Some work like pedometers, measuring your body movements, and some measure both movements and body heat. Some can be hidden, clipped onto a waistband or bra, while others are more obvious, wrapped around your arm and, if worn to a business meeting or out on the town, might draw a little attention.

Studies show that using pedometers—especially if you set a target activity level for the day—significantly boosts people's physical activity, leading to a decrease in body mass and, important for some, blood pressure.

Pedometers and other gadgets can range from $50 to a few hundred dollars. Some synch with your computer and have online and smartphone-based food logs and other tools to help you lose weight. Others have fewer add-ons.

I've used a few TDEE-measuring gadgets. I've even used two on the same day, to see if there was much discrepancy between the methods. (There wasn't—the armband estimated I burned about 75 calories more than the clip-on device.) Your mileage might vary, but here are some thoughts if you're thinking of buying one.

The pedometer-type TDEE devices, which clip to your waistband or bra, are the most office- and life-friendly option, because no one has to know you're wearing one. The one caveat is that unless you're attentive to the fact the device is clipped to your clothing, it can fall off. And because it's small—about the size of a house key—you likely won't notice it's gone. I've lost mine at a garden center, when I was loading mulch, and it's fallen off in the bathroom numerous times. You also need to be careful not to send it through the wash with your clothes.

These also are the most straightforward when it comes to checking the readouts: just look at the numbers when you click the buttons on the front. The calorie-burn estimate appears to be accurate. If you want to get extra credit for your weight-training workouts, some of the devices require you to synch them to your computer (or use a smartphone app) to input your workouts separately.

TRY THIS!

Wearing a pedometer became popular a decade ago when health officials urged everyone to try to take 10,000 steps a day. That level of activity is in line with the recommendation that for maintaining health, everyone should engage in 30 minutes of moderate activity. University studies show that taking 10,000 steps daily helps lose both weight and inches.

The armband type of TDEE measurement devices can include an optional watch, so you can more easily keep track of your numbers as the day progresses. It uses a wider variety of information. Beyond movement and steps, it also measures skin and muscle temperature as well as moisture (or sweat). That extra information is helpful in calculating your true calorie burn.

Depending on your job and how you plan to use the device, this one can be trickier to conceal, if that's an issue for you. Some people use them just for their workouts. This one is much less apt to get lost and need replacing. Also, it's fun—and motivating—to watch the calories increase over the day, and especially over the course of a workout, pushing you to work a bit harder.

These also can synch to computers and have smartphone apps that enable you to input information and keep a food diary.

Using either of these devices is a great way to motivate yourself to be active, especially if you set a target level for movement every day. Studies show that using such devices can help people increase their activity level by 26 percent a day—a tremendous boost to your NEAT calories.

Burning NEAT Calories

Let's get back to those NEAT calories. Studies show NEAT accounts from anywhere between 15 to 50 percent of your total calorie burn every day. That's either very few—or a whole heck of a lot—of calories!

A wide range of factors play into how many calories you burn as you go about the business of living your daily life. Your age, gender, weight, body composition, and perhaps even your genes govern can impact your rate of NEAT.

Some of it can be chalked up to your natural disposition—maybe you fidget a lot, don't sit still for long periods of time, have more active hobbies, and simply tend to move more than others during the course of a day. Or maybe you're more deliberate in your actions and conserve your energy, preferring quieter, less-dynamic activities.

Or maybe you have a more active job than others—carpenters burn more calories, obviously, than someone who sits at a desk all day. It only makes sense that those of us who move more get to eat more without gaining weight. It might not seem fair, but again, it's the math.

What if you, by virtue of your job, don't have as much opportunity to move around? Make opportunities! When I had an office job, whenever appropriate I'd walk to someone's office to ask a question rather than pick up the phone and call. I'd go to the supply closet myself to grab a notebook or pen, or take the stairs to a meeting. Sometimes I'd just stand up at my desk to work.

TRY THIS!

You might get some funny looks from your co-workers, but if your workplace environment allows it, set a (very quiet) alarm to go off every 30 to 60 minutes to remind you to get up and stretch.

If your workplace environment is conducive, when you have a one-on-one meeting with someone, see if you can make it a walking meeting. That way you can work and move at the same time.

Now that I'm a personal trainer, most of the people I train come to me half-wrecked with muscle imbalances from sitting at a desk all day: weak abs, tight shoulders, weak chests and thighs, stiff knees, and aching lower backs. I also remember the shoulder and hip pain I used to get from long days at the office—another reason I occasionally used to stand up while working. Your body will thank you if you get up and move more, not only by burning more calories but also by having fewer sitting-related aches and pains.

Outside of work, you might find that while dieting, it's helpful to be more active not just to burn calories but also to change your habits so you aren't tempted to snack. For many people, snacking in front of the TV has become an evening wind-down ritual. Maybe instead, doing something more active will keep your mind off snacking until you break that habit. Playing the piano or guitar or organizing a closet burns more calories than sitting in front of TV—and so does going to bed early for a little snuggling!

Beyond the weight-loss benefits of moving more, some compelling new studies are showing the importance of being active throughout the day. Even if you exercise every single day, if you spend several hours a day sedentary—especially sitting down—that lack of movement is considered a health risk, increasing your chances of developing heart disease or diabetes. Studies also show that if you spend a lot of time sitting and actually do develop one of those diseases, your chances of having a positive outcome from the effects of the disease are diminished.

Ready to take a lap around the house? Good!

Lifting to Lose

When most people first begin working out to lose weight, they generally focus on cardio workouts—exercises that use the body's biggest muscles in a repetitive fashion, which raise the heart rate and increase the flow of oxygen through the body, burning calories. Walking, running, the elliptical machine, and cardio classes all count here. If you are of a certain age, you might think of those kinds of exercise as "aerobics."

I'm suggesting a slightly different approach. I'm suggesting we focus first on weights.

Don't get me wrong: cardio workouts are fantastic, and not only for burning calories and stored fat. They also do amazing things for your health like helping with blood pressure, insulin sensitivity, and cholesterol levels. I get to all that in the next chapter. In this chapter, I suggest we first focus on weight (or strength and resistance) workouts, which also carry a variety of health benefits.

Why Weights?

Weight training, when performed in a specific format, packs a one-two punch when it comes to fat loss. Punch number one: because muscle is more metabolically active than fat, it burns more calories at rest, so the more muscle you have, the bigger your calorie furnace. That's pretty cool (or hot, as the case might be). The calorie burn difference isn't huge, but every little bit helps.

Punch number two: specifically formatted (that is, intense) weight-training workouts boost fat loss because for hours after you finish working out, your body continues to burn calories at a faster-than-normal rate. (Your body does the same thing following intense cardio workouts, which I explain in Chapter 7.)

That fat-burning boost is called the *EPOC* effect—or *excess postexercise oxygen consumption*. Basically, when you exercise with intensity, your body's systems get a little out of whack. Your heart rate goes up, your heating/cooling system has to work over-time, you sweat more, your blood pressure has to adjust, and more. After you finish working out, your body has to work over-time to return its systems to normal—and all that extra work burns more calories. Depending on the workout, the EPOC effect can last from 15 minutes to 48 hours.

 DEFINITION

Excess postexercise oxygen consumption (EPOC) is the energy your body uses after an intense workout to return to its pre-exercise state. A number of body mechanisms are responsible for boosting your metabolism during this postexercise phase, among them, replacing oxygen and fuel to your muscles and organs; removing waste from your muscles; and returning your breathing, blood circulation, and body temp back to normal.

I like to think of weight-training workouts as investments in your future: you're earning interest on your workouts through calories burned into the future. How awesome is that?

Not so awesome is a survival trick women's bodies have. (Men seem to have escaped this bit of unfairness.) Studies show intense exercise can boost women's calorie intake. Women's bodies apparently have a mechanism that self-adjusts, causing them to eat more after intense workouts to match their fuel intake to their energy output.

Women, on days you work out hard, be sure you pay extra attention to your portion sizes and food choices. I always tell my clients to drink extra water on intense workout days and, if they get stomach-growlingly hungry, to eat a little extra protein to tide them over.

If the words *intense* and *workouts* coupled together make you twitch in fear, no worries. *Intensity* is a relative term depending on your current level of strength, fitness, and health. For some, doing an incline push-up (with your hands on the wall or a weight bench) might be intense. For others, the push-up might turn into a decline push-up, with your hands on the floor and your feet elevated on a bench.

The Health Benefits of Lifting Weights

Lifting weights does a whole lot more for your body than just burn calories and tone your muscles. The health benefits are pretty amazing, and studies are continuing to show the power of picking things up and putting things down.

Resistance training can help lower your heart rate, in a good way. Weight lifting, especially the kind outlined in this chapter, can increase the efficiency of your heart, help lower your cholesterol, and improve your body's sensitivity to insulin, which can help ward off diabetes.

Weight training also helps build strong bones—an important factor as we age, helping combat osteopenia and osteoporosis. It combats age-related *sarcopenia*, or muscle loss, too. In addition, it helps improve your body composition, giving you a healthier ratio of muscle to fat.

 DEFINITION

> **Sarcopenia** is age-related muscle loss, and it starts when people are in their 30s at a rate of about 3 to 5 percent. It really starts accelerating when in the late 60s and early 70s, so the more muscle you can pack on before you hit your retirement years, the better. You'll be stronger and as a result more active, and you'll keep your metabolism firing because muscle burns more calories at rest than fat.

Not only that, but weight training can improve your posture, kick up your confidence, and give you a mood-boosting rush of endorphins (nature's painkiller). Plus, as the weight comes off, you'll have some nice, toned muscles to show off.

Have I convinced you yet? Next time you're at the gym, throw back your shoulders, walk past the lineup of cardio machines, and step into the weight room! It's not as scary as you might think—and chances are, you'll walk out feeling pretty pumped up.

Workout Sequencing

The workouts included in this book are specifically devised to work every major muscle group to not only tone your body and burn calories while doing the workouts, but also boost your EPOC. These workouts utilize a technique called *PHA*, or *peripheral heart action*.

DEFINITION

Peripheral heart action (PHA) workouts constantly change the muscle group being targeted. By shifting focus from one body part to another, your body is not only busy lifting weights, it's also busy moving fuel—blood—from one body part to the next. That extra demand on your body increases your fat burning as well as your overall fitness and level of conditioning.

PHA training burns more calories while simultaneously toning muscles. Practically speaking, it's also a great way to squeeze in a total-body workout in short period of time.

What's cool about PHA workouts is that they can be adjusted for everyone from beginners to the super advanced. All you need to change is the load, or the amount of weight lifted, and the speed at which you move from one exercise to the next.

Less-conditioned people or new exercisers should lift lighter weights and take longer breaks between exercises. Advanced exercisers should lift heavy weights and take minimal breaks, except between the circuits.

How Much Should You Lift?

Even though these workouts are designed to help you burn fat, you should still choose challenging weight loads. Opt for the heaviest you can lift while still performing the exercise with good form on the final repetition. If you're able to fling the weights around with ease (and important note: you should never fling a weight—that's a recipe for injury!) or aren't feeling very challenged at the end of a set, lift heavier weights next time!

Women often should grab heavier dumbbells from the weight rack than they do—those 3- and 5-pounders aren't going to get the results you ladies want. And just as often, men need to pick slightly lighter weights in order to maintain proper form and avoid injury.

If you're worried about building bulky muscles, stop. These workouts are not bodybuilding workouts and do not have you lifting the kind of weights necessary to gain significant muscle, although you likely will notice increased definition. Generally speaking, building muscles requires eating to support muscle building (as in, eating more than you're burning), and if you follow the diet plan in this book, that's not going to happen. Not even if you feel like you're lifting super-heavy weights.

A special note to women who feel like the legs of their jeans are getting tighter when they first start lifting weights, and are worried they are building thunder thighs: you're not. Your legs might be slightly bigger, but it's not because you're building muscle. Instead, your legs are adjusting to weight training. Sometimes when we work our legs harder than normal, the muscles retain water as part of the recovery process. Wait a day or two and that swelling will go down!

When Should You Lift?

When it comes to getting muscle definition, it's important to take rest days between your weight workouts, even if you're doing PHA training. Resting between workouts is important because when you lift weights, you're (slightly) damaging your muscles. It's during the repair process that the good stuff—the toning—happens.

So be sure you take 48 hours off between weight-training workouts so your muscles have time to adequately recover. This is especially important if you're experiencing a postworkout soreness.

TRY THIS!

As always, before starting a workout program, it's important to get your doctor's approval. If a movement causes pain, don't do it; just move to the next exercise.

The Workouts

You can do these workouts at home or at a gym. If you're lifting at home, you'll need light to moderate dumbbells ranging from 5 pounds to 25 or 30 pounds; a step or platform that, when your foot is fully placed on it, has your knee at a 90-degree angle; and resistance tubing set up so you can perform a pull-down with it.

With all the workouts, perform each circuit three times through, doing grouped exercises together back-to-back with as little time between exercises as possible. After reaching the final exercise in the circuit, take a 60-second break before completing the circuit again.

Use weights that are as heavy as you can safely handle with good form. These are not meant to be easy "light" circuits.

If you're doing these exercises at a gym and someone jumps in and uses your equipment, try to find another exercise that mimics the same movement pattern.

Warm Up

At the beginning of each workout, be sure you adequately warm up. Here's a simple routine to get your muscles ready to roll:

20 reps of bodyweight squats

10 push-ups (your choice: on wall or on floor from knees or toes)

10 reverse lunges each side (no weights)

Workout 1

Here's what to do:

Circuit 1:

> 15 walking lunges each side (intermediate and advanced: hold dumbbells)
>
> 12 lat pull-downs
>
> 12 push-ups

Circuit 2:

> 1 minute step-ups on beach, each side, keeping one foot on bench at all times (intermediate and advanced: hold weights)
>
> 12 standing overhead presses with dumbbells or barbell
>
> 12 biceps curls
>
> 12 triceps cable press-downs (or if you don't have a cable machine, perform an overhead dumbbell extension)

Circuit 3:

> 25 crunches
>
> 30 seconds bicycles (lie on your back, bringing your knee to your opposite elbow)
>
> 30 to 90 seconds planks

Workout 2

Here's what to do:

Circuit 1:

> 10 barbell or dumbbell squats
>
> 10 overhead dumbbell presses
>
> 10 cable rows (or dumbbell one-arm rows if no cable machine is available)

Circuit 2:

> 10 barbell or dumbbell reverse lunges each side
>
> 10 underhand grip pull-downs
>
> 10 incline dumbbell chest presses

Bonus round:

> 10 treadmill incline "sprints" 30 seconds each, resting 60 to 90 seconds between each sprint by lowering both the treadmill's incline and speed

TRY THIS!

If you're not comfortable running on a treadmill, the sprints can be bouts of fast walking or walking on an incline. And if you don't have a treadmill, you can do this on almost any piece of cardio equipment. Alternate "hard" and "easy" intervals.

Workout 3

Here's what to do:

Circuit 1:

> 10 stationary lunges each side
>
> 15 lat pull-downs
>
> 15 side raises

Circuit 2:

> 10 side lunges each side
>
> 10 one-arm dumbbell rows
>
> 10 flat bench dumbbell chest presses

Circuit 3:

12 biceps dumbbell curls

12 bench triceps dips

10 planks with shoulder tap each side (in plank, touch your left hand to your right shoulder and then your right hand to your left shoulder, switching sides, holding your hips steady)

Cutting Calories with Cardio

When you enter most gyms, the first thing you generally see is a long line of shiny, quietly purring cardio machines: treadmills, ellipticals, stairclimbers, bicycles, and more. We've invented dozens of ways to keep our bodies moving and sweating without ever going anywhere physically. But wellness- and weight-loss-wise, we're really going places. Cardio workouts—repetitive movements of your large muscles designed to get and keep your heart rate up—not only help you lose fat, but also come with a variety of health benefits.

Cardio machines are placed near the entrance of most gyms because they sell gym memberships. When most people initially think about starting a workout regimen, cardio workouts are the first thing that comes to mind. It's a good thought, because as I covered in the last two chapters, the more you move, the more calories you burn.

This chapter explores how and why cardio works, looks at some of the myths behind cardiovascular workouts, and offers some ways to make them more effective and less boring.

Live Longer with Cardio

Before you start moving, let's take a few seconds to look at three huge reasons, from a health standpoint, you should do cardio workouts:

- Cardio lowers your risk of premature death from all causes, and specifically from heart disease, the number-one cause of death in the United States.
- Cardio reduces your risk of death from all causes.
- Cardio gives you a higher chance of remaining active during other times of your day, reducing the health risks associated with being sedentary, as described in Chapter 5.

Drilling a little deeper, here are some more specific health-related benefits of cardio workouts:

- Lower blood pressure
- Improved cholesterol levels (cardio helps two ways, first by boosting "good" HDL cholesterol and then by lowering "bad" LDL cholesterol)
- Less body fat (including the killer intrabdominal fat, which surrounds organs and carries a slew of health risks)
- Improved insulin sensitivity (and lower risk of type 2 diabetes as a result)
- Reduced risk of blood clots

In addition to cutting risk from cardiovascular disease and diabetes, increased activity and fitness levels are linked to the following:

- Lower risks of bone fractures related to osteoporosis
- Fewer incidences of colon and breast cancer
- Reduced risk of gallbladder disease

Studies show that cardio workouts also help improve quality of life. As you age, being cardiovascularly fit helps you remain independent, reduces your risk of falls and injuries, and can be therapeutic for older people suffering from chronic illnesses. All age groups benefit from a decrease in anxiety and depression, as well as an improved sense of well-being, all thanks to cardio.

Looking at all that, why *wouldn't* you want to squeeze some cardio into your life? Less risk of death from all causes and a more positive outlook on life? Sign me up!

How Much Cardio Do You Need?

Chances are you've heard varying reports about exactly how much cardio you need to do. It can be hard to sort the facts from the fiction. I'm a personal trainer, and even I get frustrated with the various recommendations!

My rule of thumb: when it comes to the facts, if in doubt, go to the experts—those who spend time in labs working with real people and real data. They generally have better information than an infomercial fitness model or someone selling the latest workout program.

TRY THIS!

If what you're about to read freaks you out, hang on! Just think back to the EPOC effect I explained in the last chapter. And remember, some exercise is always better than no exercise.

Experts from the American College of Sports Medicine, who pretty much set the standard for all things exercise, came up with the following findings.

To prevent weight gain and, perhaps, experience some modest weight loss, engage in moderate-intensity exercise for 150 to 250 minutes a week (bottom range: 30 minutes 5 times a week; top range: 50 minutes 5 times a week). If you're trying to lose weight and engaging in this amount of exercise, it's going to be especially important to also follow a diet program that moderately restricts calorie intake—like the one in this book!

To lose a significant amount of weight—and, once the weight is off, improve the chance of keeping it off—studies show getting more than 250 minutes of physical activity a week is optimum.

In other words, trying to exercise for an hour or more most days of the week helps you lose weight and also improves your chances for keeping it off.

All-Out or Nothing?

Now for a pep talk. If that hour a day seems like it's just too much and you're wondering why you even bother trying (a story I hear all too frequently), first of all, stop talking to yourself like that.

Remember, *any* exercise is better than *no* exercise. Get what exercise you can, when you can. Fitting activities into the nooks and crannies of your day counts. Plus, I'll show you strategies for making this happen. And good news: the resistance training workouts in the previous chapter are formatted in such a way to count toward those minutes!

TRY THIS!

Break your workouts into separate sessions—say, 15 minutes at lunch or 45 minutes after work. It all adds up!

You might have noticed the words *moderate intensity* in the preceding section. What exactly is moderate intensity? And what if you work out harder than "moderately"? You'd have to work out for less time, that's what!

How do you know how hard you're working—whether it registers as "moderate intensity" or not? There are many ways of calculating levels of exertion, but I'm all for keeping it simple. Let's stick with two easy ways: perceived exertion and heart rate.

Perceived Exertion

Perceived exertion is your own assessment of how hard you're working. A fancy scale called the Borg scale measures exertion on a scale to 1 to 20, but that's a wide range of numbers to try to sort through. We're all about keeping it simple. Here's my easy version:

Level 1: Sitting on the couch, watching your favorite TV show.

Level 2: A happy little Sunday stroll in the park— little effort, feeling great!

Level 3: This takes that stroll and turns it into a more purposeful walk—the pace is a little faster, and you're breathing harder, but you're still comfortable.

Level 4: That walk? It's like you're going up little hill. You start to sweat, but you feel good and can talk with no problem.

Level 5: This is where it starts to turn into work— the hill is steeper, and the pace is quicker. You're sweating more, and you wouldn't say you're exactly comfortable, but you can still carry on a conversation fairly easily.

Level 6:	That conversation? It's more like a series of short answers. You're feeling slightly breathless, and your sweat level kicks up.
Level 7:	You don't want to talk, but you can. And you know you're going to need a shower later because you're sweating ... a lot.
Level 8:	No words. Only grunts. When will this end?
Level 9:	I'm afraid I'm going to keel over.
Level 10:	I keeled over!

Using this scale, low intensity, great for warming up and for beginners or those coming back to exercise after a layoff, is levels 3 or 4. Moderate intensity is levels 5 or 6. High intensity, great for more advanced people to burn more calories, is levels 7 or 8.

Heart Rate

Your heart rate is the most honest method of checking your intensity. When I say "most honest," it's a reality check we all can use sometimes to see if we're slacking off a little, pushing too hard, or working just hard enough.

You can measure your heart rate using an old-school method by counting your heart beats via pulse points, usually your wrist or your neck, or more new school with a heart-rate monitor. Some cardio machines come equipped with monitors, or you can buy one for $30 or up, depending on how many options you choose. If you buy a heart-rate monitor, get one that has a band that wraps around your chest for the most accurate results. If you do buy a monitor, it doesn't have to be fancy (although fancy can be fun). Mostly, you just want the monitor to count your heartbeats. You don't need the alarms and fitness tests that come on some higher-priced models.

TRY THIS!

To take your pulse, use a light touch so you don't affect your finding, especially on your neck. For your wrist, lightly place two fingers just above your thumb. Take it for 15 seconds, multiply by 4, and that's your heart rate. Or you can check your pulse on your carotid artery (your neck), just to the side of your larynx. Be sure to only lightly press.

How do you figure your cardio working zone using your heart rate? By doing some more math! There are many formulas, but let's look at a very basic one to get you rolling.

First, you need to determine your estimated maximum heart rate (MHR).

$$220 - \text{your age} = \text{MHR}$$

Now, here are the zones, based on your heart rate:

Zone 1: Low intensity, 60 to 70 percent of your MHR (MHR × 0.6 to MHR × 0.7)

Zone 2: Moderate intensity, 70 to 80 percent of your MHR (MHR × 0.7 to MHR × 0.8)

Zone 3: High intensity, 80 to 90 percent of your MHR (MHR × 0.8 to MHR × 0.9)

Let's say you're 35 years old. That gives you an MHR of 185 (220 – your age). Your heart rate zones would be as follows:

Low intensity: 111 to 130 (185 × 0.6 and 185 × 0.7)

Moderate intensity: 130 to 148 (185 × 0.7 and 185 × 0.8)

High intensity: 148 to 167 (185 × 0.8 and
185 × 0.9)

Depending on your fitness level, you should work within the appropriate zone. How do you know what zone is appropriate for you? A lot of that has to do with your fitness history and current level of fitness.

Remember: what's considered "low intensity" for one person might be all-out effort for another. We're all a little different, so as I tell my clients, keep your eyes on your own papers! Don't pay attention to everyone else—do *your* workout, at *your* level, especially if you're just starting a new program.

 DANGER ZONE

Some medications, notably beta blockers, calcium-channel blockers, nitrates, diuretics, bronchodilators, vasodilators, and antidepressants, can impact your heart rate, making it beat faster or slower than normal. If you're taking prescription medication, check with your pharmacist to see whether it might impact your heart rate.

If you haven't worked out in the past few months, concentrate on low-intensity workouts (zone 1) and gradually work up your endurance (how long you can work out) and intensity (how hard/fast you can go), moving into the moderate-intensity zone 2 workouts.

If you're already in pretty good shape, start at zone 2 and occasionally push your intensity into zone 3.

I'll outline some workouts later that help you do this through metabolic training and interval workouts.

When to Work Out

You might have heard that for optimum results, you have to do your cardio first thing in the morning, as soon as you get out of bed, on an empty stomach. The theory was that early morning cardio burns more stored fat because your fuel tank is already on empty when you wake up.

Studies show that might not be the case—that having some fuel in your system before you work out actually enables you to work out harder and longer, burning even more calories in the long run.

My opinion on timing? It has to be practical. If you love early morning cardio on an empty stomach, do it. I have clients who can't work out in the morning after eating breakfast—they feel nauseated. And I have other clients who feel dizzy if they don't eat first. Do what fits your schedule, your body, and your lifestyle.

It's true that clients who work out first thing in the morning tend to be more regular exercisers because they get their workouts done early, before the occasional problems that arise during the course of a day throw them off-course. But does it matter? No, not at all. Do what works for you—the important thing is that you do something!

Work Out!

One of the major complaints about cardio workouts is that they're boring. Let's look at some ways to make them not-so-boring.

Studies show that working out with motivating music cuts your perceived exertion and lets you work out longer. So if you're planning on a straight-up 45-minute elliptical session, listen to some music you love to get more out of it.

And mix it up. I'm a fan of cardio machine circuits. If you have access to a few different machines, make a little round of them. Start on the elliptical, move to the stairs or rowing machine, then the bike, then the treadmill. You'll sweat more than ever as your body works to adapt to the different movements—and your workout will fly by!

TRY THIS!

When it comes to cardio, be adventurous. Try a new class, join a recreation league sports team (volleyball? masters swimming? softball?), learn ballroom dancing, or go for a weekend hike. Constantly doing new activities means your body is constantly adapting to new movements, burning more calories. Plus, it's fun!

Take a class or pop in an exercise DVD. Not only will you get a great workout, but chances are you'll work your body in a variety of planes of motion, working different muscles and boosting the effectiveness even more.

Intervals! Incorporate these into your workouts. Basically, warm up for 5 to 10 minutes and then alternate intervals of hard work with easier "recovery" work. These intervals can range in length from 30 seconds to 2 minutes.

The beauty of intervals is that almost anyone, no matter what fitness level, can do them. They're also a great way to get into shape fast because they employ the EPOC concept (remember that from the last chapter?). For the very unconditioned, interval training might mean alternating slow treadmill walking with slightly faster treadmill walking. For the super fit, it can mean alternating jogging on a flat treadmill with sprints at a 10 percent incline. Because you know you have a break coming up, you're able to work harder, boosting your overall workload, fitness, *and* calorie burn.

Finally, try a metabolic conditioning circuit. This one is my absolute favorite. I'm including two versions in the following sections, one using a cardio machine and one without, so you can get it done no matter where you are! Either way, you're going to end up a hot, sweaty mess—but with a metabolism that's chugging along at a good clip, burning calories like crazy!

Dreadmill Delivery

For some reason, this workout became nicknamed "Kamikaze Session." It uses cardio equipment and light weights. Warm up on the cardio equipment of your choice and then pick four or five conditioning exercises and rotate through them before getting on the machine again.

A moderately intense workout could look like this:

> 5 minutes on the elliptical machine to warm up
>
> 20 reverse lunges
>
> 10 jumping jacks
>
> 20 kettlebell or dumbbell swings
>
> 15 push-ups with your hands on the floor or a bench
>
> 15 biceps curls
>
> 15 triceps bench dips
>
> 20 crunches

Then, hop back on the cardio equipment, and alternate 1 minute each of easy and challenging intervals. Then get back off the machine and go through the circuit again. Repeat until 20 to 30 minutes have passed, ending always with an easy bout on the cardio machine, allowing your heart rate to return to near-normal. By the third time through, you'll be drenched in sweat and feeling an endorphin rush.

TRY THIS!

Buddy up! Having a friend keep you company during a cardio workout can help push you to work harder because when you're tempted to slack, your friend will be there to urge you on. And even better, when you're done, you can congratulate each other on a job well done. My clients who work out in groups get the best results!

Metabolic "Playlist" Circuit

This is a challenging but fun workout and is a good one to do with a buddy. What I especially like about it is that you can work through it at your own pace. The fitter you are, the faster you can move from exercise to exercise. Be sure to pace yourself, especially if it's been a while since you've worked out.

Grab your MP3 player, and make a playlist with seven peppy songs you love, each in the 3:30- to 4-minute range.

Warm up with a brisk walk. Then push "play" and do each of the following circuits for the length of the song, repeating until the song has ended. When the next song starts, move on to the next circuit.

Song 1:

> 10 bodyweight squats
>
> 10 push-ups (your hands on a bench or the floor)
>
> 10 Russian twists (each side)
>
> 10-second rest

Song 2:

10 lunges each leg (do all reps on one leg before switching to the other leg)

1 plank walk each direction (get into plank position and "walk" your arms and legs 5 steps in each direction)

10 ab bicycles each side (lie on your back, reach your elbow to your opposite knee)

10-second rest

Song 3:

15 jumping jacks

10 side lunges, alternating sides

10 plank shoulder taps each side (in plank, touch your left hand to your right shoulder and then your right hand to your left shoulder, switching sides)

10-second rest

Song 4:

10 squats to kick each side, switching sides

10 twisting planks (in plank position, lift your left arm up until it reaches toward ceiling and then switch to your other side, alternating sides)

10 crunches

10-second rest

Song 5:

> 10 jump squats
>
> 10 "spiderman" planks (in plank position, bring your elbow to your knee, alternating sides)
>
> 5 inchworms (remaining in plank, walk your hands toward your feet and then back out, keeping your feet stationary)
>
> 10-second rest

Song 6:

> 15 seal jacks (just like a jumping jack except instead of going side to side, go to the front, clapping your arms in front of your chest, your feet scissoring front to back)
>
> 10 mountain climbers each side (your hands on a bench if necessary)
>
> 10 curtsy lunges (like a lunge, except curtsy!), switching sides
>
> 10-second rest

Song 7:

> 10 gate swings (hop your legs out into a wide squat and then back to the middle in a narrow squat, slow and steady)
>
> 5 push-ups
>
> 10 v-ups (lying flat on your back on the floor, arms extended overhead, simultaneously raise your arms, torso, and legs so your body forms a V; if this is too challenging, do regular crunches)
>
> 10-second rest

Sample Week

Here's an easy way to schedule your workouts to get the most from your time in the gym:

Monday:	Resistance training circuit (Chapter 6), 15 minutes on elliptical using the interval technique
Tuesday:	Kamikaze workout
Wednesday:	Resistance training circuit
Thursday:	Steady-state cardio, 45 to 60 minutes
Friday:	Resistance training workout, 15 minutes on elliptical
Saturday:	Optional Metabolic "Playlist" Circuit
Sunday:	Off

If you feel overly tired or sore, take an extra rest day to allow your muscles to recover. And be sure to drink plenty of water!

Making It Work

So now you know what you're supposed to eat and when you're supposed to eat it. You understand how to calculate the number of calories you burn in a day and how to increase that number by moving your body more and incorporating exercise into your life. And you have your "whys"—the reasons you're embarking on this weight-loss journey in the first place—all in order.

Now you're like all the people who join the gym New Year's Day. Except—lucky you!—you're not like all those people who give up the gym after a few weeks because you'll still be following your program and watching the pounds melt off for months. Why? Because you have a secret weapon—this book!—which will help you stay on-plan until you reach your goals.

In this chapter, I give you some coaching and tips to help you stay on track. My plan is for you to still be following this plan 2 months from now as you cross the finish line and reach your goal. And maybe even develop some new habits that will last a lifetime!

When the Honeymoon's Over

Chances are, the first few days of your new program are going to feel great. You might experience a craving or two, you might feel a little tired, and you might experience some muscle soreness from your workouts. But your motivation will be high. It might even—dare I say it?—be fun!

It's after the first week or so that the enthusiasm can start to wane. If that happens to you, know this is perfectly normal, you're right on track, and we've all been there. When work or home issues start to flare up, when the novelty fades, when you're tired and haven't had the best day ever, it's tempting to start to cheat a little bit on your diet or skip a workout or two.

How can you avoid that? How can you keep going even when you feel like you really don't want to?

The good news is—and this is strictly anecdotal—it seems that for most of my clients, just when they're at their breaking point and in need of a pep talk, they suddenly have a major break-through on the scale or with the measuring tape!

Planning for Setbacks

Willpower alone doesn't cut it when it comes to maintaining a diet or other lifestyle change. It just doesn't have the power to sustain you. Contrary to popular belief, the keys to sticking with a program long term have very little to do with "getting tough" and "sucking it up." The inevitable challenges arise not because you're weak or somehow can't get it together.

What does have the power to sustain you and keep you going when the going gets tough? Your beliefs—your mind's core operating system—trump willpower every time. When your beliefs start to change—when you see that you *can* stick with a diet, that you *do* have control over your behavior, and that you *can* be successful—things fall into place. Your beliefs all stem from your whys. When you uncover the gut-level realization about *why* you want to lose weight, things tend to line up a little more.

When your willpower starts to fade, remember that you really *do* want to keep going. Look back at the whys you explored in Chapter 1. Are they the real reason(s) you want to lose weight? Or have you found some others along the way? Look at the motivational pictures you clipped—that's why you clipped them in the first place, to remind you why you're doing this. Talk to your support crew, and let them know how you feel and that you're struggling a bit.

Also know that life is going to get in the way sometimes. It's a fact. Some days you'll be tired. Some days a last-minute issue will pop up and test your commitment. Expect it to happen. In fact, *plan* for it to happen.

It's how you handle those problems that determines whether you're successful with your weight-loss plan or not.

 TRY THIS!

We wouldn't be in the middle of an obesity epidemic if dieting was easy. When the going gets tough, rather than focusing on external motivations like how you look or what the scale says, try focusing on larger ideals, such as your health and self-care or having more energy to devote to your family. Remember: you're worth the effort!

Sometimes diet slip-ups happen as a result of being on autopilot and not recognizing hazards when they arise. This has happened to me: every Thursday night, I would end up sneaking a trip through the drive-thru or making a quick, not-so-healthy food choice for my final meal of the day. And every time I did, I would scold myself, and yet the next week I would go through the same routine.

That continued until I finally took a couple minutes to actually think about what was going on that led to me making the same choice week after week. It had nothing to do with willpower. It was simply a scheduling problem I had to fix. A work commitment meant my normal eating pattern was thrown off, making me hungry, plus I got out of work late Thursday nights after leading a tough cardio class. Adding to all that, on Thursdays I also was out of all my prepared food. Talk about a perfect storm for not-so-healthy eating! After I added a mid-afternoon snack and made sure I had some good and healthy food at home to look forward to, the drive-thru visits ended.

The moral of the story: if you find that you're hitting walls when it comes to sticking with the program, take some time to explore the reasons behind it—and then do something about it.

Like me, chances are your little struggles and problems have nothing to do with your willpower. They're just problems you haven't yet identified. Maybe it's a logistics issue like mine, or maybe you need to shift your beliefs a bit and come up with a solution.

Two Types of Hunger

The biggest area of struggle, and the most important weight-loss-wise, is the diet. Getting your diet under control is the number-one indicator of weight-loss success. Again, it comes down to that math problem, calories in versus calories out.

The next time you feel like straying outside the boundaries of your eating plan, ask yourself: *Am I really hungry? Or do I just want to eat?* How can you tell the difference? Let's look at some ways to differentiate between the two.

Physical Versus Emotional Hunger

Physical hunger comes on slowly, usually 3 hours or so after the last time you ate. It's generally accompanied by a rumbling or growling stomach.

Even though physical hunger is genuine hunger, you usually can wait a little while to eat. And then after you *do* eat, you feel satisfied and the hunger goes away. Fortunately for most people reading this book, we rarely experience true physical hunger, so when it happens, it's kind of a surprise.

Emotional hunger, on the other hand, tends to come on quickly, regardless of the last time you ate. It wants to be fed, and fed *now*. Usually, it wants a specific kind of food like chips, pizza, cookies, or chocolate—generally not salad or chicken—and won't be satisfied until it has that food. And even then, it's not really satisfied.

Another clue you're dealing with emotional hunger: after you eat, you might feel a little guilty about it, and that guilt might make you want to give up your diet and eat even more. Maybe you'll restart again tomorrow, or maybe not until Monday.

When you're dieting, occasionally you will feel a stomach rumble or two indicating you're physically hungry. We're all wired differently, but it only makes sense that creating a calorie deficit—cutting back on the fuel your body uses to power it so it uses stored fuel instead—makes some people feel actual hunger. That hunger shouldn't give you a stomachache, keep you up at night, or cause any disruption in your life. But a little mild hunger between meals? It's to be expected. If you're following the plan, chances are you've got a meal coming right up to help curb it.

Combating Emotional Eating

Entire books have been written about emotional eating—why we do it; how to stop it; the links between our food and our culture, religion, belief system, and family; etc. I'm not going to get into all that, because basically, it always comes back to creating that all-important calorie deficit. Our emotions matter, but they shouldn't dictate all our behaviors.

Emotional eating doesn't only happen when you're having a bad day or are feeling down about something. It also happens around happy occasions and celebrations. What do you do if you earn a pay raise or a promotion? You go out to dinner to celebrate. Seeing long-lost family and friends? It's time for a celebratory feast! Weddings, birthdays, even funerals—each usually features a lavish spread of food and drink.

Here are some common emotional eating triggers, both positive and negative:

- Stress
- Boredom
- Loneliness
- Visiting friends
- Ladies' time of the month
- The smell or sight of food
- Seeing other people eat
- Time of day
- Habit
- Watching television
- Going to the movies
- Someone cooked/baked you food
- Financial problems
- Relationship problems
- Parties and holidays
- Feeling unloved, unworthy, overwhelmed, or frustrated
- Anger
- Fatigue
- Being at a restaurant or buffet

Do any of these situations look familiar? Chances are you can add even more to the list. Did you come up with a few more personal triggers?

> **TRY THIS!**
>
> Next time you feel compelled to eat between meals, take some time to think about what's going on to fuel that compulsion and see if you can make some changes to avoid those feelings. It can be uncomfortable, but knowing what makes you tick is the key to not only taking off the weight, but also keeping it off.

Isn't it at least a little comforting to know that you're normal in having those triggers? The trick is to come up with strategies to deal with anything that might spark cravings *before* they arise. That way, if you know Aunt Sarah is going to try to goad you into having a big slice of her homemade raspberry pie at Sunday dinner, you're prepared.

Food Is Fuel

I'm not going to get all crazy and say that food is only energy (although, truthfully, it is) because it also can be far more than that. But when it comes right down to it, healthy and fit people generally look at food as either fuel to power your body and brain as you live your life, or your body's building blocks (remember: you are what you eat!) that supply it with much-needed vitamins and minerals to create health and vitality.

Changing your behavior, your mind-set, and your eating patterns will take time. In the meanwhile, here are some things you can do instead of eating:

- Drink some water. And then some more water.
- Organize a drawer.
- Chew some gum.
- Brew a cup of tea.
- Browse fitness-related websites for added motivation.
- Play a musical instrument.
- Go shopping (anywhere that doesn't sell food!).

- Get a pedicure or manicure.
- Play a video game (preferably one that requires you to get up off the couch).
- Plan a home- or apartment-improvement project.
- Go for a walk.
- Create a blog to document your progress.
- Learn a craft.
- Take a nap or go to bed early.

Notice a trend? Most of those things keep your hands busy so they don't have time to transport food to your mouth.

But if no matter what you do, you just can't get the idea of eating out of your head, munch on something low in calories. Want some crunch? Baby carrots and celery sticks are more diet-friendly than chips. Something creamy? Fat-free plain Greek yogurt with fruit is a more waistline-friendly choice than ice cream. Or chop up a banana, put it in a plastic container, and pop it in the freezer for a couple hours. When it's frozen, blend it in the food processor—it will taste almost like ice cream!

Doing It Anyway

This is where the "get tough" part enters the picture. Some days you're not going to feel like working out. Go do it anyway, even if you don't want to do it! A little while into the workout, you probably will feel a lot better about it.

We all have days when we don't want to exercise—just as we have days when we don't feel like going to work, brushing our teeth, or making the bed. But we do those things anyway, right? Even people who make their living in the fitness industry occasionally lack motivation. That's when you have to make your own motivation!

Again, the internet can be a good source of inspiration. So can watching feel-good sports movies—*Rocky*, *Step Up*, *Rudy*, *Hoosiers*,

Flashdance, Blue Crush, Elektra, Without Limits, or whatever your go-to pick-me-up movie is. The list of motivational movie contenders is long (and often, there's a good deal of motivating eye candy to keep your interest!).

> **TRY THIS!**
>
> The next time you're tempted to skip a workout because you're tired and stressed, make yourself work out for 15 minutes anyway. If at the end of 15 minutes you still aren't into it, you can quit for the day. But most likely, you'll feel better and keep going.

Another trick some people use to stay on track is a reward-and-penalty system. Most of us are motivated when it comes to thinking of things to reward ourselves with if we hit a particular benchmark, such as a number on the scale or an inch loss. It's best if the reward isn't food related. Maybe go to a movie or buy a new gadget or outfit as a reward, for example.

But don't stop there. What's even more effective is if you add another layer to this agreement with yourself—a layer of penalty if you don't follow through. So not only do you *not* earn a reward, you actually *lose* something if you miss the mark. It's sort of like being grounded when you were a kid. That isn't so much fun to think about, is it?

What's a realistic penalty you could enforce upon yourself if you fail on your plan? Maybe not being able to go to a party or do something fun you've been looking forward to. Some people will force themselves to donate money to a cause or political candidate they don't support. Penalties can be even more motivating than rewards!

Staying on the Wagon

When it comes to sticking with any diet and workout plan, it's easier to stay on the wagon than it is to keep crawling back on after you fall off. Inertia has a way of setting in if you skip several workouts in a row. You can begin to forget how great you felt when you made it to the gym (or the basement, or the park, or wherever you work out), and you can come up with a dozen reasons why you shouldn't work out.

Same thing with your diet—that energized feeling you get from fueling your body with just the right amount of the right foods? It's exhilarating! But it's also easy to forget that feeling when you've been loading up on not-so-healthy foods.

Get back on that wagon! And this time, do your best not to fall off! Your fitness mojo will come back in a couple days.

Staying Social

You're not going to be hiding under a rock for the duration of this plan—at least I hope you're not! You've got to have some strategies for negotiating life in the real world: going out to eat, socializing with family and friends, while avoiding what for some of us is the inevitable array of birthday cakes and open candy dishes at work.

Sometimes when we start to make changes in our lives like working out or eating different foods, those around us can appear to be less than supportive, while others rally to help. In this chapter, we explore some ways to deal with the naysayers—and maybe even help them in the process.

In Chapter 2, I discussed assembling a support crew to help you stay on track. With some people, however, it's best to employ what I call the "shock and awe" approach—don't involve them in what you're doing differently in your life. Let your results speak for themselves. But more on that later.

Eating Out

We eat out a lot—in fact, one out of every five meals Americans consume is eaten at a restaurant, according to the National Restaurant Association. It's just not realistic to think that for the duration of your diet, you're going to avoid eating out entirely. But still, that's a whole lot of meals not to be in control of during the course of a week.

Take Control

The trick to successfully eating out without it impacting your waistline is to take as much control as possible of the situation before you step foot into the restaurant. Remember: you're in charge!

First, there's your mind-set. Most of us look at eating out as something special, an occasion. Plus, there's the buffet effect I talked about earlier—when presented with a variety of food, we instantly want to eat more. It's human nature. But no matter which way you look at it, those meals eaten outside your house are still just meals, and it's important to treat them that way. A meal is a meal is a meal—just another opportunity to fuel your body with nutrition to help you attain your desired result.

Beyond controlling your mind-set, what can you do before you go out so the meal doesn't turn into a fat-laden fiasco? You have to think ahead! As always, forewarned is forearmed. Go to the restaurant with a specific plan in mind, just as you do every other meal you eat.

Whenever possible, try to look at the menu beforehand. You usually can do this online, and many chain eateries also offer a nutritional breakdown of menu items on their websites. In fact, the National Restaurant Association reports that as of 2012, 36 percent of Americans have used the internet to research nutrition information before going out to eat.

Order Up!

Sometimes, though, even the healthiest choice on a restaurant menu leaves a lot to be desired. But that doesn't mean you're out of luck.

I used to be hesitant when it came to making special requests at restaurants. That changed one day when I got into trouble with a waiter at one of my usual hangouts.

I was having lunch with a business associate when the waiter came over to chat with us. We were regulars, after all, which helps in these situations. I mentioned how I wished I could order buffalo wings (hey, personal trainers like 'em, too!), but I didn't want them to be breaded and fried and loaded with fat and calories. The waiter looked at me like I was an idiot. "Why don't you just order grilled chicken with the buffalo sauce?"

Well, duh! It had never occurred to me I could order it that way! After being soundly lectured to order whatever I wanted and let the kitchen deal with it, I started to become a little more adventurous in my ordering.

In fact, I even have an unofficial breakfast item at a local diner—the Wendy Bowl, a mix of oatmeal, scrambled egg whites, strawberries, and a teaspoon of peanut butter. Stop making that face—it's good! It really is!

 TRY THIS!

Tell your server you're on a diet, and ask him or her if they can make a recommendation about good choices to order. Every time I've done this, I've been met with nothing but support. Some restaurants even have separate smart-choice menus for those on special diets, but the waitstaff doesn't offer them unless you ask.

The trick to successful custom ordering is to be aware of your surroundings and to seek your waitperson's help. Let him or her know you're on a special eating plan.

More importantly, if the restaurant is experiencing a rush and there's a long line of folks waiting to get in, don't throw a bunch of strange requests at your server because that's just asking for trouble. Keep it as simple as possible. And always ask for special orders kindly—and leave a good tip!

More Dining-Out-on-a-Diet Tips

Here are some tried-and-true tips for eating out:

If smaller, lunch-size portions are available, order those because you'll be less tempted to overeat. Otherwise, get a to-go box along with your meal, and as soon as your food arrives, divide your meal and box half of it for later. You'll eat less, and you'll have a meal for later you won't have to prepare.

Also, stick with proteins and veggies, if possible. It's harder to control how starches like pasta, potatoes, and rice are cooked and whether they contain butter or other calorie- or fat-laden flavors. Instead, ask if you can replace that starchy side dish with a second veggie side.

Order your veggies grilled or steamed and without any butter. Many times veggies come slathered in a buttery sauce. You don't need that.

Opt for grilled or broiled fish, poultry, seafood, beef, and other proteins. And it doesn't hurt to specify that you'd like them with no fat added during or after cooking. You know how succulent and juicy some cuts of meat look when they arrive at the table? That's because some chefs dot them with a pat of butter as soon as they're done cooking.

Beware the salad bar! It's tempting to think the salad bar is your best bet, but be on high alert as you approach it. The fresh vegetables are obviously low-calorie options, but be careful of prepared salads like pasta, potato, or any creamy-dressed concoctions because they likely contain excess fat and even sugar. Before you add cottage cheese to your plate from the salad bar, ask your server if it's full- or low-fat. Why bother? Because there's a 100-calorie—or more—difference between a cup of low-fat and regular cottage cheese.

TRY THIS!

Did you ever notice that after a restaurant meal, you feel especially interested in enjoying dessert? There's something about the added flavors in restaurant entrées that makes some diners crave sweets. Drink extra water to fill you up, and ward off any temptation!

Dealing with Family

This is where the going can get especially tricky. It can be hard for some people to allow their family and friends to change because they might unconsciously regard your decision to lose weight or get in shape as a threat to your relationship with them. Really.

Some of my training clients have told me that their family—both spouses and children—complained about the time they spent in the gym, or wondered why they suddenly had to go about making all these changes in their lives when everything was just fine the way it used to be.

This is where a little calm reassurance comes into play. Maybe you need to have a one-on-one with your spouse to let him or her know the reasons you're working out or losing weight— namely, not to get in shape so you can attract someone new! Be as genuine as possible in your explanation. Are you doing this so you'll have more energy, confidence, and improved health? Is it to show off a hot bod at your upcoming high school reunion? Or is it to look great for your partner while you're on vacation together? With time, your spouse will likely come around and should actually encourage your efforts to lose weight and get into shape. Maybe he or she will even join you!

Including your children as much as possible in the changes you're making is a great way to get them on board and help establish in them healthy habits that will last a lifetime. Children emulate what they see, so if they see you being active and eating healthfully, they're more apt to do the same as they mature. Get them involved with food prep if they are old enough. They also will appreciate the time you spend with them being active together. Some of my best childhood memories of my father come from the evening walks we used to take together.

Socializing on a Diet

Again, forewarned is forearmed. Before you get together with friends and family, whether for a simple dinner, a night out, a holiday, or a party, go with a plan in place. This is especially important if your gatherings—whether with friends or extended family—tend to revolve around food and drink.

When you're attending a gathering, bring healthy options both for yourself and for sharing. I find it's best to not advertise that the food is "healthy." Be a little sneaky, and try to come up with options that aren't necessarily obvious like the old standard veggie and fruit platter, which is bound to bring at least one "rabbit food" comment. Many great resources are available in print and online for fun and healthy appetizers. Try baked chicken tenders, shrimp, melon wrapped in prosciutto—get creative!

Keep in mind that you are in control of both the situation and what you put in your mouth, even if you're in the presence of family members who like to think they're in control. Remember that *you* are the boss of you, even if Aunt Sarah is dead-set on you eating that slice of homemade raspberry pie. Choosing not to eat it doesn't mean you're choosing not to love her. It simply means you're choosing not to eat pie.

TRY THIS!

Have a healthy, filling snack like a piece of fruit, some veggies, or a meal from your meal plan before you go to a food-related gathering. That way, you'll be less tempted to indulge!

It's also surprisingly common to encounter criticism when you're dieting. People might make fun of your food choices; tell you you're looking frail, sick, or tired; or express concern that you're "taking this whole diet and exercise thing too far." It's ironic that some people are quicker to make a negative comment when you eat salad than when you mow through half a pizza. It's also a shame.

Chances are, that criticism is prompted by guilt or defensiveness. It's easier for someone feeling defensive to poke holes in what you're doing rather than change what they're doing—even if you have no intention of changing them or judging their food choices.

Don't take these comments personally. In the moment, especially if you're still new with your diet, it can be hard to shrug off such comments, but try to let them go. As someone whose mere presence inspires guilt, I know this can be tough. I've had people actually turn around and go the other way at the grocery store when they see me coming down the aisle! Some days I think this is funny. Some days, frankly, it's not so funny.

The naysayers are the ones you're going to shock and awe, as I discussed earlier. Make a firm decision not to discuss your diet or your workouts with them. When you're excited about something, it can be hard not to talk about it, but it's none of their business. And besides, you don't need their approval or their opinion. Instead, let your results do your talking for you. It'll be fun to see their reaction the next time they see you looking slimmer and trimmer.

But be realistic. If that skirmish with Aunt Sarah over the raspberry pie threatens to turn into an outright battle, take the piece of pie. Tell her you're going to eat it later, so you can really enjoy it, and box it up. Then either give it away or throw it out later. Perhaps it's not the most honest thing to do, but sometimes you have to do what you have to do to keep the peace. A piece of pie isn't worth getting into an argument over.

TRY THIS!

Next time someone insists you try their delicious food, ask for a raincheck—or for the recipe—because you'd love to try it another time.

When you stick with your plan and people start seeing results, you're likely going to inspire your family and friends to make changes in their own lives.

Livin' Large

Going out for an evening on the town? You can have fun and not totally blow all the hard work you've put in over the previous week. As discussed earlier, it doesn't take much to undo a calorie deficit, especially if you're close to reaching your goal or are generally smaller to begin with.

Keep in mind that if you have a drink or two of alcohol, you become less inhibited, and that's a major threat to your diet. I'm not worried about you dancing on a table—that's your own business, although you definitely could burn off some major calories! I am concerned about what those drinks, and lowered inhibitions, can do to your food choices and intake.

When you've had a few drinks, you start to feel invincible, and for some of us, that can mean we care a little less about the consequences of our actions. Among other things, that makes us more apt to eat foods we normally would avoid—chips, pizza, cookies, or a fat-laden, late-night after-party breakfast. Those extra calories definitely won't help your diet. No one is saying you shouldn't have fun. The key point is to not let what you drink affect what you eat.

DANGER ZONE

Remember, beverages contain calories, too! In fact, even though alcohol technically falls in the carbohydrate category, 1 gram alcohol contains 7 calories, as opposed to the 4 calories per gram protein and other carbohydrates. And fruit juices can contain a lot of calories, so be careful there.

Here are some ways to indulge in adult beverages without causing too much damage to your diet:

- Alternate alcoholic drinks with water to save calories. This helps you stay hydrated so you feel great tomorrow morning, too. Best bet: start with the water so you feel full before you ever take a sip of alcohol.

- Choose wine, light beer, or cocktails made with low- to no-calorie mixers such as club soda, water, sugar-free syrups, and low-calorie juices. Wine spritzers have always been a great choice.

- Skip the mixer and try a flavored liquor on the rocks instead. A variety of flavor-infused liquors are available, with flavors ranging from fruit and chocolate to jalapeño peppers, all with no extra calories.

So go out, have fun, and enjoy yourself! And the next morning, wake up feeling great about all those calories you burned on the dance floor, instead of filled with regret about any excess calories you ate!

Working It at Work

Years ago I worked in an office where everyone's birthday was celebrated in grand style—cake, ice cream, soda, the whole she-bang. It's nice that people cared enough about each other to have parties, but after a while, it got to be too much. I didn't want to be a party pooper, but at the same time, I and some of my co-workers didn't want to eat a bunch of sugary food and end up feeling bloated and headachy later. So we found ourselves scheduling meetings outside the office whenever we knew a party was going to be held, no offense meant to the birthday boy or girl.

If something similar happens in your office and it's starting to affect your waistline, you can still attend the birthday gathering but politely decline a piece of cake, scoop of ice cream, and a sugary soda. Carry a water glass into the break room with you so you can say, "No, thanks. I have my water," when offered something not on your diet plan. And be sure to sing out loudly during the birthday song!

As for the ubiquitous candy jar—that's a tough one. Having a stash of healthy food in your desk for emergencies is always a good idea. A 100-calorie snack-size packet of almonds, for example, can tide you over in the midst of a craving. At lunch, opt for a foil pouch of tuna—another low-calorie option that contains lots of protein to help keep you feeling satiated throughout the afternoon.

If you're someone who has a mid-afternoon sweets craving, look for individually packaged low-calorie dark chocolate squares, and limit yourself to just one a day.

Final Week Countdown

If you're losing weight for a specific event like a wedding, reunion, or some other special occasion, this chapter will help get you picture-perfect for the big day. In the following pages, I show you how to fine-tune your diet to help you appear leaner, and I also offer some suggestions for modifying your workouts slightly to boost that leanness quotient to the next level.

The little adjustments I introduce here are simply meant to help flatten your stomach by eliminating bloating, ensure your digestive system is humming along, and also help you feel trimmer when the big day arrives by boosting your calorie burn.

These last-chance tweaks are optional and, although perfectly safe, aren't meant to be followed long-term. Don't think because they're "last chance," they're necessarily any better, more advanced, or more effective than what's outlined in the diet and workout plans earlier in the book. Think of them as occasional boosters when you need a little more *oomph*.

Hello, H₂O

We're going to get a little personal now—we're going to talk about your trips to the bathroom. Believe it or not, what happens when you're in there is a good indicator of what's going on with your body in general.

It also plays a role in aesthetics, like how flat your belly is and whether you're retaining water, which can cause bloating and swollen ankles.

Got Water?

One of the most important things you can do to avoid stomach bloating (and keep your skin looking fresh!) is to drink at least six to eight glasses of water a day—work up to a gallon if you can. This is especially important when you're amping up your workouts.

How do you know if you're drinking enough water? Here's a good indicator: when you go to the bathroom to urinate, the toilet water should be pale yellow, like diluted lemonade. If it's darker and you haven't taken a vitamin containing riboflavin (vitamin B_2)—which is notorious for giving you neon-yellow urine—in the past few hours, you need to drink more water.

If you never seem to remember to drink enough water, keep this image in mind: have you ever given a droopy houseplant a thorough dousing of water and watched it come back to life? Its stems and leaves swell before your eyes, and the plant transforms from wilted and sad to vital and healthy in a matter of minutes. Now imagine that's your body every time you take a drink. Who wouldn't want to feel vital and healthy all the time?

Why is drinking water so important? It might sound contradictory, but drinking too little water can actually cause your body to retain water, causing your soft tissues—including your muscles, tendons, fascia, and skin—to swell. It's vital to ensure you're keeping your body hydrated and happy by giving it a good drink several times a day.

TRY THIS!

Some studies have shown that drinking water helps speed
your metabolism, boosting weight loss slightly. Drinking
2 cups of water before every meal was shown to help
middle-age and older dieters lose more weight—and keep
it off!

Flush the Fat

Another thing to keep in mind: where, exactly, does fat go
when you lose it? Does it just melt or disappear? No, neither.
Remember, fat is simply the stored energy your body has been
tapping into as you've created a calorie deficit to help you lose
weight. What happens when you burn something? It creates
waste, right?

Your body gets rid of the waste by sweating it out (water!), by
urination (again, water!), and also via your lungs when you
breathe (adequate hydration plays a key role here, too). Drinking
water helps flush out all that burned-up fat. So drink up!

DANGER ZONE

Even though this chapter emphasizes adequate water
consumption, it's important to know that you can drink *too
much* water, although it's rare. A condition called dilutional
hyponatremia, or "water intoxication," has occurred in
marathon runners and other endurance athletes who chug
too much water during an event. It happens when the
kidneys get overloaded with water and can't process it,
leading to a bunch of other potentially dangerous problems.
Everyone's water needs are different, but if you don't exceed
1 gallon a day and are healthy, you're safe. When in doubt,
ask your doctor.

Speaking of flushing, if you've been following the diet plan up until now, you're getting plenty of fiber to help avoid constipation. However, even if your fiber intake is where it should be—for women under age 50, that's 25 grams daily; for women over 50, 21 grams; for men under 50, it's 38 grams; for men over 50, 30 grams—drinking too little water can cause your digestion to come to a halt.

Guzzle that water, because the more you keep things moving through your digestive system, the flatter your stomach will appear and, even more importantly, the better you'll feel.

Tips for a Flat Belly

In addition to getting plenty of water, there are other things you can do to flatten your midsection.

Limiting Certain Foods

It seems a little convoluted, but following a weight-loss-friendly diet can actually cause your stomach to bloat. All those healthy, nutrient-rich, fiber-rich, stomach-filling vegetables you've been eating, especially the cruciferous veggies like broccoli and cauliflower, can make you feel gassy and a little rounder in the belly. It's a little disconcerting and potentially embarrassing. Flatulence, unless you're in junior high, is never cool.

A few days before your event, start weaning off the gas-causing veggies, and focus more on vegetables that don't cause as much gas. Green beans, asparagus, and spinach are fantastic choices. They tend to be a little easier for your system to process.

Another bloat- and gas-causing culprit is legumes, which include any of the dried bean family such as black beans, kidney beans, cannelloni beans, etc. Temporarily cut back on the beans to help tighten up your tummy.

For this week, try trimming your consumption of wheat products like bread, pasta, and cereal because these products can cause some stomach swelling in certain people. It's a little trendy right now to eliminate wheat, but I'm not suggesting you cut it entirely from your diet forever. Just try easing away from it for a few days and see if it helps flatten your belly and eliminate bloating.

Another food group to temporarily reduce in your diet is dairy. Some people have a harder time processing dairy products than others. They get gas, which causes their stomach to swell a bit. Yogurt, because of its lower lactose levels, is often the best tolerated of the dairy products, and the probiotics it contains actually can be helpful with digestion in some people.

 DANGER ZONE

Remember the earlier discussion about how some people eliminate entire food groups rather than watch their caloric intake and portion sizes when they diet? Don't do that! Even though you're temporarily cutting back on some specific foods here, it's not reasonable or even healthy to do it forever. (A diagnosed food allergy or sensitivity is, of course, the exception.) When in doubt, check with your doctor.

If you've been eating or drinking low-sugar food products and beverages that contain sugar alcohols, eliminate them because they can cause bloating and some very sudden gas effects in some people. Look for words like *xylitol, sorbitol, maltitol,* and *glycerol* on the package labels of the foods you've been eating. You also can tell by looking at the nutrition facts on product labels. Sugar alcohols are usually listed there. Some people aren't affected by them at all, and some of the sugar alcohols have more gas-causing effects than others. If you've been noticing a trend in that area, it's worth a little investigation.

Other belly-bloating culprits include anything that causes you to swallow air, like chewing gum, which can contain sugar alcohols to make them taste sweet without adding sugar, or eating too fast. Carbonated "fizzy" drinks also can contribute to the effect.

It's also a good idea to watch your sodium intake. There's no need to go crazy and eliminate it completely, and if you've been following the diet in this book, chances are your sodium intake is well within an optimal range. Even so, watch your use of salt-laden spice blends and, obviously, the salt shaker.

Sodium can cause your body to hold water and swell. This affects not only your stomach, but also your ankles and soft tissues.

Increasing Certain Foods

Now on to the happier portion of this last-minute plan: what you get to eat and add to the plan to help boost its stomach-flattening effects!

When it comes to your starchy carbs, you want to think about foods that are easy for your system to digest, like rice, white potatoes, and sweet potatoes. These foods help keep your stomach flat. Because they're not as fibrous as some other choices, it's more important than ever to be sure your water intake is optimal. (Yes, again with the water.) As you're following along with your normal food plan, start swapping out your starchy choices and see if it makes a difference.

Also opt for high-water-content fruits and veggies like watermelon, celery, onions, and cucumbers. They'll keep you feeling full as well as contribute to hydration.

When it comes to flushing out your system—or helping it get rid of water—grapefruit and pineapple are yummy fruits that also serve as natural diuretics.

DANGER ZONE

Grapefruit and some herbs can interact with some prescription drugs. If you're on prescription medication, check with your pharmacist before you add grapefruit or herbs to your diet.

Some herbal teas also have diuretic and stomach-flattening qualities. Try dandelion, peppermint, and ginger, either hot or cold. Several major tea companies package blends of herbs and fruits together to create teas that not only taste great but also can help your body naturally flush itself out.

When shopping for an herbal tea blend, look for the word *detox* on the label. Also double-check the ingredients to ensure it's filled with the right herbs for you and not simply a laxative that will have you spending a lot of time in the bathroom. Senna is a popular ingredient in laxative herbal teas, so unless you need to get things moving, choose another teas without senna.

Burn It Off!

Now it's time to refine your workouts and kick them up a few notches. One word describes these changes: *sweatastic!* I'm going to make you sweat … and then sweat some more! I hope you're ready (insert evil chuckle here).

For this final week, we're going to get a little radical, and you're going to feel like a bona fide athlete when you're done. I promise. This last-minute plan includes a 7-day countdown of workouts, ramping up the workouts you've already been doing to optimize their efficiency.

This is not the time to forget your water bottle when you go to the gym. (Yes, I'm a broken record when it comes to water consumption, but it's really that important.)

Day 1

Do either the Dreadmill Delivery or Metabolic "Playlist" Circuit from Chapter 7.

Add 10 minutes of extra steady-state (moderate-intensity, no intervals) cardio at the end, if you have time, so your workout lasts for about 45 to 60 minutes.

Cool down completely by allowing your heart rate to return to normal before hitting the shower.

If you have time, at some other point during the day, go for a 30-minute walk.

Day 2

Pick one of the resistance-training workouts in Chapter 6. Warm up as always, and go through the exercises as usual—except add a 2- or 3-minute cardio burst between circuits, when you'd normally be resting. You won't be sitting around at all during this workout! Move, move, move!

Between circuits, perform a conditioning exercise like jumping rope, jumping jacks, or kettlebell swings. Or jog in place, do step-ups on a bench—anything. Just keep moving!

If you're afraid of creating a spectacle in the gym, get on the elliptical or another piece of cardio equipment for the 2- or 3-minute time span and really go for it. Really get your heart rate up, and then, when 2 or 3 minutes have passed, go through the circuit again.

Good news: you only have to do each circuit twice.

TRY THIS!

If you choose Workout 1, skip the cardio between the ab exercises at the final circuit, but instead go through the circuit twice, with no break.

Finish with 15 to 20 minutes of steady-state (moderate-intensity, no intervals) cardio before cooling down and allowing your heart rate to return to normal. Then, take a shower—you're going to need it.

Day 3

Repeat Day 1, with either the Dreadmill Delivery or Metabolic "Playlist" Circuit from Chapter 7.

Add 10 minutes of extra steady-state (moderate-intensity, no intervals) cardio at the end, if you have time, so your workout lasts for about 45 to 60 minutes.

Again, cool down completely before hitting the shower. If you have time earlier or later in the day, take another walk.

Day 4

Repeat Day 1, using a different resistance-training circuit than you have been using.

Look at today as your last-chance workout. Tomorrow, you lower the intensity.

You're almost there!

Day 5

It's all steady-state from here. You're going to lower your workload so you're working at a moderate intensity for the entire workout.

You can spend 45 to 60 minutes on a piece of cardio equipment, do a low-impact cardio class, or perform the cardio machine circuit outlined in Chapter 7. Do whatever feels right for you today.

You've worked hard so far this week, and today is a day to just cruise along and bask in your accomplishments.

Day 6

Repeat Day 5, except this time, add a little more intensity, with a few intervals thrown in to keep things interesting.

You don't need to get crazy with these intervals—every couple minutes or so, increase your speed, the resistance on the cardio equipment, or the incline at which you're working to get your heart and breathing rates up a little. Then back off. Throw in five or six intervals during the course of the workout.

Day 7

Go for a nice long walk or easy bike ride for 45 to 60 minutes. You're just keeping your muscles loose and your blood pumping here—and giving you a healthy dose of those all-important mood-boosting and stress-busting endorphins.

When time's up, pat yourself on the back. Congratulations— you've made it to the finish line! Now, go grab a drink of water.

Easy Does It!

You might notice you're down an extra few pounds at the end of this final week, thanks to the changes in your diet and workout intensity. This is a good news/bad news situation. Don't expect that extra bit of weight loss to last long because it likely can be attributed to water weight loss. Yes, even after all my harping on drinking water, that's part of the deal.

You might be tempted to party it up at the end of the week—especially if you were targeting your diet for a specific event or vacation and the end of the plan coincides with the event. Don't be surprised, should you happen to indulge in an adult beverage or two, if you feel the effects of the alcohol a little more than normal, thanks to that water weight loss.

The next chapter details how to get off the diet without regaining all the weight, but for now, enjoy your success, and go (a little) easy on the fun stuff!

Keeping the Weight Off

You've worked your butt off—literally!—to get to your goal, and you've made it. Congratulations!

Even with the best support crew, a sensible diet, and a kick-butt workout plan, losing weight takes discipline, self-development, and hard work—and no one can get that work done but *you*. And you did it. Give yourself a pat on the back for making it to the finish line. You deserve it!

The sobering news is that even though you've made it to the end, this is really only the beginning. Or maybe, better, a new beginning to a brand-new phase called "maintenance." Maintenance is probably the most challenging phase of weight loss.

Within a few years of reaching their goals, the vast majority of dieters eventually regain the weight they've lost. Even experts seem confounded by how to help people keep off the weight. The statistics paint a pretty dismal picture: depending on the source, experts estimate anywhere from 66 to 80 percent put the weight back on. That's a lot of pounds to regain and a lot of people facing another set of "before" pictures. Let's see what we can do to put you in the 20 to 33 percent that does keep the weight off—for good!

A New Normal

It's going to take more than a diet mind-set to help you keep off the weight. We've already established that you have discipline, just by virtue of the fact you've made it to your goal. Now you're going to put that discipline to further use, but in a way that lets you live an exceptional life.

We need to define a new normal, because "normal" everyday life is what put you in the position of wanting to lose weight in the first place, right?

I want you to picture future you—that's you 2 months, 1 year, or 5 years from now. Is future you thinking about embarking on another weight-loss plan? Or is future you feeling fit and energetic, thanks to some decisions present you—you, right now, today—made?

You're going to retool and customize your program so you can maintain your weight loss for a lifetime—so future you looks a lot like present you. This will take some patience and experimentation to find what works for you. Again, we're all different, with different priorities, schedules, goals, and lifestyles, which means this will be a learning process.

Developing an Exit Strategy

When my clients go on weight-loss diets, I stress to them the importance of having an exit strategy—a specific plan to get off the diet and back to "normal" eating. The truth is, most clients ignore me when I start my "exit strategy" speech and think what I'm telling them doesn't apply to them because they are somehow different. Or they don't understand what I'm talking about until they're in the middle of a postdiet meltdown.

I put the word "normal" in quotes for a reason. I'm not talking about how my clients normally ate before they went on the diet—not at all. Again, that "normal" eating pattern is what got them to the point where they ended up wanting to lose weight. Although "normal" eating might be comfortable and fun, it's not productive or even, likely, very healthy.

This new normal isn't the "normal" American diet either. With our raging obesity epidemic, eating like a normal American won't keep you trim. According to the U.S. Centers for Disease Control and Prevention, based on their *body mass index* (*BMI*), 34 percent of adults over the age of 20 are considered overweight. Another 34 percent are in the obese category. Put those numbers together, and that's a staggering 68 percent of adults who are above "normal" weight.

 DEFINITION

> The **body mass index** (**BMI**) is a calculation that takes into consideration height and weight. It's not an accurate measurement for bodybuilders or those with a lot of muscle, but it's a good starting point in assessing health risk due to weight. Adults with a BMI between 25 and 29.9 are considered overweight; adults with BMI of 30 or higher are considered obese.

When it comes to younger Americans, 18 percent aged 12 to 19 are obese, and 19 percent of children aged 6 to 11 also fall into the obese category.

Obviously, we need to redefine "normal" eating. And that's the challenge. It requires eating outside the norm, and for some of us, that's uncomfortable.

I vote you go for exceptional—the shock-and-awe effect I talked about in Chapter 9. You can choose a vital, healthy life brimming with energy and fun.

The first step: even though you've been following a "diet," let's stop using that word. Now that you've reached the finish line, you no longer need to be on lockdown. But that doesn't mean you should engage in a series of feeding frenzies.

Finding that balance between "dieting" and exercising portion control to keep your weight in check is a challenge, and unless you're mentally prepared and have a specific plan in place, you're likely going to experience a pretty specific series of events.

What (Usually) Happens When the Diet Ends

Here's a pretty typical scenario of what happens when you (and when I say "you," I mean people in general) go off a diet:

Stage 1: This stage occurs the first couple days after you meet your goal. You have a well-deserved treat (or two or three), generally a food you haven't enjoyed for a while and that's long been among your favorites.

You back off your workouts, taking some rest days. That's okay, and even encouraged, because it's important to occasionally take recovery time when you're been working out regularly.

Even with the added treats and reduction in activity, you feel great, and you're surprised you're able to get away with all this without immediately swelling up or seeing a huge change on the scale.

Stage 2: You continue to indulge in treats, but you notice something strange. It's almost as if your body is trying to make up for all the treats you didn't have while you were dieting. Whereas before, one or two cookies were enough, now you can scarf down a lot more than that and still want more.

Even with all the cravings and indulgences, you're feeling pretty invincible. What's more, the scale barely reflects the extra calories you're taking in.

You start up your workouts again, but the truth is, without the urgency of your old goal, your intensity goes down a little.

Stage 3: Oops. How did *that* happen? Your jeans aren't zipping up anymore, or if they are, you have to go through a series of deep knee bends to stretch them out so you can walk normally, and you're forced to wear a loose shirt so the resulting muffin top/spare tire doesn't show.

You know you've got to get this under control, and soon. Tomorrow, in fact. But tonight, you'll just have a final pizza, or piece of cake, or fettuccine Alfredo, or maybe all three ….

TRY THIS!

When you reach the diet finish line, continue to weigh yourself at regular intervals. Continue to drink plenty of water to keep yourself feeling full, too.

Stage 4: Darn it. It's been a while since you've stepped on the scale, but here you are, and it's worse than you thought. You're just about back to square one. Do you really want to go through all this again? Ugh.

Confession: I know these stages intimately, because I've not only witnessed my clients go through them, I've experienced them myself. And from my own experience, I can tell you the exit strategy is the most important part of the weight-loss process.

Transitioning to Maintenance Mode

So how do you transition yourself from weight-loss to maintenance mode? Slowly, that's how. It's also important to understand that some of your urge to overindulge after a diet might be physiological and not because you're somehow mentally weak (again, one of the stories we tell ourselves).

Some experts believe our bodies have a natural set-point weight—a weight your body "likes" to weigh—and until your body adjusts to its new weight, it will fight like crazy to go back to its former set point. Others blame hormones.

The fact that we don't know why it happens is irrelevant. What is relevant is that you do something about it, right?

Redefining *Normal*

This is where the discipline comes in, starting as soon as you hit your goal. Yes, enjoy some treats, but then get right back on that exceptional-eating wagon. Future you—the one in stages 3 and 4—will be grateful.

First of all, you need to keep working out. That much has been established. Not surprisingly, experts can't seem to agree on exactly how much you need to work out to maintain your weight. The American Council on Sports Medicine, in its most recent position stand, said there's not enough data yet to support making recommendations about how much physical activity is necessary to prevent people from regaining lost weight.

Likewise, the *Journal of the American Medical Association* published a study that showed that women who successfully maintained normal weight (gaining 5 pounds or less) over the course of 13 years averaged about 1 hour of moderate-intensity activity a day. But other experts wondered if those results were applicable to everyone.

Let's look at the habits of people who have successfully kept off their weight after losing it. Since 1994, the National Weight Control Registry (NWRC) has been tracking people who have maintained significant weight loss. The group relies on surveys, questionnaires, and self-reports of more than 10,000 people who have lost significant amounts of weight—and more importantly, especially for our purposes, who have kept the weight off.

Here are some of the NWRC's nuts-and-bolts findings:

- 78 percent of those who kept the weight off eat breakfast every day.

- 75 percent weigh themselves at least once a week, and the more often they stepped on the scale, the lower their BMI.

- 62 percent watch less than 10 hours of TV a week.

- A whopping 90 percent exercise about 1 hour a day.

It boils down to this: to be exceptional, you have to eat regularly, stay active, exercise, and keep track of your weight. Sounds like it just takes some common sense, doesn't it?

Even if the experts can't agree about making a blanket statement about how much exercise is necessary to maintain weight loss, from a commonsense perspective, it comes back to creating a balance between your TDEE (the number of calories you burn in a day) and how many calories you take in. (Remember that discussion from Chapter 5?)

TRY THIS!

Keep your workouts fun during maintenance. Don't make them all about burning calories. Instead, try new things to enjoy exercise for its own sake. Take a yoga class, try jazz dance, golf (leave the cart at the clubhouse!), or maybe even challenge yourself to become even fitter by signing up for a 5k or 10k race. This will help prevent boredom and keep you inspired.

I propose that during maintenance mode, devices like pedometers and the other calorie-burn-estimating gadgets can be even more important than during weight-loss mode. There's much less guesswork involved in hitting the proper calorie mark when using these devices because you have data to work with.

If, for example, your body burns 1,800 calories in an average day (like mine does), that's how many calories you get to eat to maintain your weight (like I do).

Do I wish my body burned more calories than that on a regular basis? Yes! But the fact is, it doesn't burn more than that and so that's my everyday-normal-walking-around calorie target. If I'm trying to tighten things up, like everyone else, I step up my workouts a little and trim my intake.

If working out for the sake of maintaining your weight isn't motivating enough, turn back to Chapter 7 and review many of the awesome health benefits of exercising like a lowered risk of dying prematurely. If that's not a motivator, what is? Your body was built to move!

Eating for a Lifetime

Creating a successful diet exit strategy takes some finesse and patience. Start by gradually increasing your portion sizes and widening your "healthy" food choices, adding some more fruit to your menu and maybe boosting the number of starchy carbs you eat slightly, still keeping them as unprocessed as possible.

Watch how your body reacts to these changes—if your weight suddenly bumps up and stays up for several days, back off the portions a little. And as always, be sure you're drinking enough water.

Allow yourself one treat a week—a planned meal where you don't worry about how many calories you're taking in, or whether you're getting a balanced number of macronutrients (protein, fat, and carbs). Just eat, and enjoy. But tread lightly here. Be sure to get back to your regular food choices immediately.

Some people find that having a treat meal sets off a feeding frenzy or outright binge. Rather than beat yourself up over this, instead, strive to get back to your regular "exceptional" eating pattern as soon as you can. Then, after the haze of the binge has passed, examine what might have happened to set it off. Use it as a learning experience!

TRY THIS!

If you have a major diet blowout and you want to get back on track, start eating sensibly in a pattern that follows the diet plan in Chapter 3. Drink water, work out, and be sure you're eating adequate veggies and protein. Your body will start to feel better almost immediately, and that should motivate you to stick with it.

Here are your key strategies to maintaining weight loss:

- Continue to eat four or five meals a day.
- Drink plenty of water.
- Watch your portion sizes, and double-check them regularly.
- Keep working out and maintaining the balance between energy in and energy out.

Changing Your Outlook

I recently spoke with a wonderful lady at my gym. She's been battling her weight for almost her entire adult life—up and down and up and down again. She's fed up with it, and also, frankly (she told me), with herself.

She told me she was afraid of making anymore changes, though, because she didn't want to make the wrong change. Along with the joint pain that comes from carrying around extra weight, she's now suffering from metabolic syndrome: diabetes, high blood pressure, high cholesterol—the whole nine yards. She's working with a panel of doctors and a nutritionist to regain control of her weight and her health.

It can be tough to know how to handle some clients because we all process information a little differently. Tough love works for some, while gentle nudges are better for others. All I could think when I looked at her was, how could she be afraid of changing her "normal" patterns of eating and exercising when they clearly weren't working for her? When they were, in fact, working *against* her in a pretty serious fashion?

We went over all that and I asked her, point blank: "Aren't you more scared of *not* changing anything?"

And that's the moment she got it. Since then, she's been making gradual lifestyle changes and is feeling great. The scale is starting to move, too.

Accepting the reality that what we view as "normal" really isn't "normal" at all can be a hard reality, but there's no way around it.

Rather than looking at weight maintenance as being held captive to the scale, look at it as a way to be free from the scourge of weight-related conditions plaguing you. Heart disease, diabetes, high blood pressure, and more are directly correlated with carrying excess body fat.

Choose to be an exception of the norm! Future you will be glad you did.

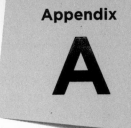
Glossary

calorie A measurement of the potential heat in foods; the amount of energy expended to raise the temperature of 1 gram water by 1 degree Celsius. There are 3,500 calories in 1 pound of weight.

clean eating Eating healthful, whole foods as close to their natural state as possible. It's trendy now, but it's how our grandparents ate.

excess postexercise oxygen consumption (EPOC) The energy your body uses after a hard workout to return to a normal, preworkout state. When you exercise hard, all of your body's systems are affected—circulation, heart rate, temperature, and more. It can take between 15 minutes and several hours for your body to return to normal, which boosts your calorie burn.

ghrelin One of the hunger hormones, among other things, ghrelin tells you when to eat. When you're tired, more of it circulates in your body, and experts theorize this could be why we sometimes overeat when we're tired.

leptin A hunger hormone, leptin lets you know when you've had enough to eat. When you're tired, less of it circulates in your body.

metabolic conditioning Metabolic workouts are designed to boost your metabolism, and as a result, your calorie burn, by increasing your EPOC. The workouts generally combine calisthenics and resistance training, either using your own body weight or free weights.

nonexercise activity thermogenesis (NEAT) The amount of energy, or number of calories, you burn over the course of a normal day, not including any calories you burn while exercising. NEAT calories play a tremendous role in regulating weight, accounting for as much as 50 percent of your energy expenditure.

perceived exertion A subjective method of measuring your workout intensity. To work out at moderate intensity, on a scale of 1 to 10, you should be at about level 5 or 6—feeling a little sweaty and still able to talk, but unable to sing.

peripheral heart action workout A training technique to boost calorie burn and general fitness by alternately working large muscle groups so your body must adapt by shifting fuel to different parts of the body.

set point theory Some experts theorize our body has a "happy" weight—or set point—at which it's comfortable. This can be why it's challenging to maintain weight loss. Some studies show regular exercise over time can help lower this "set" weight.

starchy carbohydrate Carbohydrates are generally divided into two classes: starchy and nonstarchy vegetables, based in part on how they're metabolized in the body, their nutrient density, and their fiber and sugar content. Starchy carbs contain three or more sugars, while fruits and vegetables contain one or two forms of sugar.

sugar alcohol A low-calorie artificial sweetener used in many foods. It's a form of sugar, but it doesn't cause decay. However, it might have minimal impact on blood sugar and might cause stomach bloating or gas in some individuals.

total daily energy expenditure (TDEE) The number of calories your body burns over the course of a day. To maintain your weight, you must create a balance between calorie consumption and TDEE. To lose 1 pound of weight per week, you have to eat 500 calories per day less than you burn; to lose 2 pounds per week, you have to increase that deficit to 1,000 calories a day.

The resources provided here are designed to help keep you motivated and customize the program even further. There's nothing like signing a contract to make you accountable, and I've included a sample one for you to consider.

Then, if you want, you can chart your body's changing BMI and body fat percentage using the calculations provided. You can even tailor your workouts even more by figuring your unique target heart training zones.

To start, some wonderful books and websites can help you maintain your fitness mojo. My most-recommended fitness books are *The New Rules of Lifting* series by Lou Schuler and Alwyn Cosgrove. The books are entertaining reads, and the workout programs are designed to be safe, effective, and efficient.

When it comes to sticking with a program, Tom Venuto's *The Body Fat Solution: Five Principles for Burning Fat, Building Lean Muscle, Ending Emotional Eating, and Maintaining Your Perfect Weight* can help galvanize your willpower and keep you on track.

Looking for some variety in your home workouts? DVDs can be a great option, but the sheer number of them on the market can be overwhelming. Videofitness.com is a free resource featuring DVD reviews written by real people, a fitness forum, and even a video swap.

Make a Contract with Yourself

Making a formal contract with yourself can be an effective way of boosting your diet success. To do so, first identify three key actions you're going to hold yourself accountable for during the span of the contract (2 months). These actions should be directly correlated with diet success, and they should be individual to you and the challenges you anticipate facing. Possible examples include exercising for a specific amount of time each week, preparing your meals in advance, and not letting the needs of others interfere with your commitment to yourself, as shown in the following sample contract.

And be sure someone witnesses your signature to boost your accountability factor!

Sample Contract

I, _____, commit and agree to take the following steps to increase my chances for weight-loss success. I willingly sign this agreement to improve my accountability with myself.

1. I will exercise for a minimum of 4 hours per week, working an appropriate intensity for my fitness level. I also will strive to be more active in my daily life by seeking opportunities to increase my physical activity at work and at home.

2. I will plan my meals in advance and, each night before retiring, be sure everything I need for the following day is readily accessible. When necessary, I will change my habits to avoid engaging in emotional eating.

3. I won't let a bad day interfere with my progress, and I also will not put the needs of others before my own, doing for them what they can do for themselves rather than taking care of myself. If it appears a conflict will arise, I will do my best to find a compromise before problems result so I am able to keep this commitment with myself.

_____

Name

_____

Date

_____

Witness

Calculation Station

When it comes right down to it, a lot of math is involved with weight loss. The following sections offer some formulas to help pinpoint your unique numbers.

Body Fat

Many methods of measuring your body composition are available, including bioimpedance (scales and handheld devices), fat calipers, dunk tanks, and more. You also can estimate your body fat using calculations based on your body dimensions.

Women:

Factor 1	(Weight × 0.732) + 8.987
Factor 2	Wrist (widest point) ÷ 3.140
Factor 3	Waist (naval) × 0.157
Factor 4	Hip (widest point) × 0.249
Factor 5	Forearm (fullest point) × 0.434

Lean body mass = factor 1 + factor 2 − factor 3 − factor 4 + factor 5

Body fat weight = total bodyweight − lean body mass

Body fat percentage = (body fat weight × 100) ÷ total bodyweight

Body fat percentage categories for women:

Essential fat	10 to 12 percent
Athletes	13 to 20 percent
Fitness	21 to 24 percent
Acceptable	25 to 31 percent
Obese	32 percent and above

Men:

Factor 1	(Total body weight $\times$ 1.082) + 94.42
Factor 2	Waist $\times$ 4.15

Lean body mass = factor 1 – factor 2

Body fat weight = total bodyweight – lean body mass

Body fat percentage = (body fat weight $\times$ 100) $\div$ total bodyweight

Body fat percentage categories for men:

Essential fat	2 to 5 percent
Athletes	6 to 13 percent
Fitness	14 to 17 percent
Acceptable	18 to 25 percent
Obese	26 percent and above

Body Mass Index

Health and wellness professionals often use the body mass index (BMI) to assess health risk. BMI is simply a calculation using your height and weight to estimate your weight status (underweight, normal, overweight, or obese). BMI is considered a starting-point calculation because it doesn't take into consideration body composition.

To calculate your BMI, the first thing you need to do is calculate how tall you are in inches and square that number (or multiply it by itself).

For example, if you're 5 feet, 8 inches tall, that's 68 inches, so $68 \times 68 = 4,624$. Let's call that result "h^2." And let's imagine you weigh 180 pounds. Here's how you'd calculate your BMI:

BMI = weight in pounds $\div$ $h^2 \times$ 703.0704

BMI = 180 $\div$ 4,642 $\times$ 703.0704

BMI = 27

BMI Classifications

Classification	BMI	Obesity Classification	Disease Risk*
Underweight	<18.5		Increased
Healthy weight	18.5 to 24.9		Normal
Overweight	25 to 34.9		Increased
Obese	30 to 34.9	I	High
	35 to 39.9	II	Very high
Extremely obese	>40	III	Extremely high

Disease risk refers to likelihood of developing type 2 diabetes and cardiovascular disease.

Heart Rate Training Zones

In Chapter 7, I detailed a general way of calculating your appropriate heart rate training zones to ensure you're working at the appropriate level for optimal calorie burn. To make those zones more individual to you, you can use the Karvonen Formula to calculate your unique training zones. The formula looks like this:

Training heart rate = ([MHR – resting heart rate] × desired intensity) + resting heart rate

To calculate your resting heart rate, first thing in the morning, before you get out of bed or engage in any significant movement, take your pulse for 1 full minute, starting with a count of 0. Lightly place your fingers along your carotid artery to count the number of times your heart beats. (Pressing too hard can cause your pulse to slow.)

Now, we'll figure your MHR, which is simply your age subtracted from 220. Let's say you're 35 years old—that gives you a theoretical MHR of 185 (again, 220 – 35). Your resting heart rate is 75, and you want to exercise within your moderate-intensity zone, which is zone 2, 70 to 80 percent. Remember: perform calculations inside parentheses first!

Minimum training heart rate = ([185 − 75] × 0.7) + 75

Minimum training heart zone = (110 × 0.7) + 75 = 152

Maximum training heart rate = ([185 − 75] × 0.8) + 75

Maximum training heart zone = (110 × 0.8) + 75 = 163

So to exercise at moderate intensity, you should aim to keep your heart rate between 152 and 163. (If you haven't been exercising regularly, it's a good idea to start in zone 1, or exercise within the 60 to 70 percent zone.)

Index

U–V

updating go-to meals, 40-42

vegetables
  canned, 43
  eating out tips, 100
  free, 35
  fresh in-season, 43
  frozen, 43
  gas-causing, 110
  gradually increasing, 34
  nonstarchy, 34
  prepping, 45
  serving sizes, 34
very active activity level, 54

W–X–Y–Z

warm up, 67
water
  benefits, 108-109
  daily requirement, 36
  drinking enough, 108
  drinking too much, 109
  recommendations, 108
websites
  food logs, 18
  weight-loss/fitness forums, 24
weekend treats, 11
weekly meals example, 47-50
weigh-ins
  choosing day, 3
  daily, 4
  starting point, 3-4
  weekly, 3

weight loss
  boosting, 110-113
  calorie deficits, 54-55
  equation, 9
  flat belly boost
    increasing certain foods, 112-113
    increasing workout intensity, 113-116
    limiting certain foods, 110-112
  forums, 24
  two pounds per week, 30
weight training, 62
  benefits, 63
    calorie burning, 62
    health, 63-64
  choosing weight amounts, 65-66
  EPOC effect, 62
  equipment requirements, 67
  PHA, 64-65
  resting between workouts, 66
  schedule, 85
  warm up, 67
  women's bodies survival trick, 63
  workout 1, 68
  workout 2, 68-69
  workout 3, 69-70
wheat product belly-bloat, 111
whole-grain breads, 42
women
  body survival trick, 63
  thunder thigh worries, 66
work dieting challenges, 106